T0348635

Anesthesia for Otolaryngology

Editors

ADAM I. LEVINE
SAMUEL DEMARIA Jr
SATISH GOVINDARAJ

OTOLARYNGOLOGIC CLINICS OF NORTH AMERICA

www.oto.theclinics.com

Consulting Editor
SUJANA S. CHANDRASEKHAR

December 2019 • Volume 52 • Number 6

ELSEVIER

1600 John F. Kennedy Boulevard • Suite 1800 • Philadelphia, Pennsylvania, 19103-2899

http://www.oto.theclinics.com

OTOLARYNGOLOGIC CLINICS OF NORTH AMERICA Volume 52, Number 6
December 2019 ISSN 0030-6665, ISBN-13: 978-0-323-68306-7

Editor: Stacy Eastman
Developmental Editor: Laura Kavanaugh

Otolaryngologic Clinics of North America (ISSN 0030-6665) is published bimonthly by Elsevier, Inc., 360 Park Avenue South, New York, NY 10010-1710. Months of issue are February, April, June, August, October, and December. Business and Editorial Offices: 1600 John F. Kennedy Blvd., Suite 1800, Philadelphia, PA 19103-2899. Customer Service Office: 6277 Sea Harbor Drive, Orlando, FL 32887-4800. Periodicals postage paid at New York, NY and additional mailing offices. Subscription prices are $412.00 per year (US individuals), $889.00 per year (US institutions), $100.00 per year (US student/resident), $548.00 per year (Canadian individuals), $1127.00 per year (Canadian institutions), $564.00 per year (international individuals), $1127.00 per year (international institutions), $270.00 per year (international & Canadian student/resident). Foreign air speed delivery is included in all *Clinics*' subscription prices. All prices are subject to change without notice. **POSTMASTER:** Send address changes to *Otolaryngologic Clinics of North America*, Elsevier Health Sciences Division, Subscription Customer Service, 3251 Riverport Lane, Maryland Heights, MO 63043. **Telephone: 1-800-654-2452 (U.S. and Canada); 314-447-8871 (outside U.S. and Canada). Fax: 314-447-8029. E-mail: journalscustomerservice-usa@elsevier.com (for print support); journalsonlinesupport-usa@elsevier.com (for online support).**

Reprints. For copies of 100 or more of articles in this publication, please contact the Commercial Reprints Department, Elsevier Inc., 360 Park Avenue South, New York, NY 10010-1710. Tel.: 212-633-3874; Fax: 212-633-3820; E-mail: reprints@elsevier.com.

Otolaryngologic Clinics of North America is also published in Spanish by McGraw-Hill Interamericana Editores S.A., P.O. Box 5-237, 06500 Mexico D.F., Mexico.

Otolaryngologic Clinics of North America is covered in *MEDLINE/PubMed (Index Medicus), Current Contents/Clinical Medicine, Excerpta Medica, BIOSIS, Science Citation Index,* and *ISI/BIOMED.*

Contributors

CONSULTING EDITOR

SUJANA S. CHANDRASEKHAR, MD, FACS, FAAOHNS
Past President, American Academy of Otolaryngology–Head and Neck Surgery, Secretary-Treasurer, American Otological Society, Partner, ENT & Allergy Associates, LLP, Clinical Professor, Department of Otolaryngology–Head and Neck Surgery, Donald and Barbara Zucker School of Medicine at Hofstra/Northwell, Hempstead, New York, USA; Clinical Associate Professor, Department of Otolaryngology–Head and Neck Surgery, Icahn School of Medicine at Mount Sinai, New York, New York, USA

EDITORS

ADAM I. LEVINE, MD
Professor, Departments of Anesthesiology, Perioperative and Pain Medicine, Otolaryngology–Head and Neck Surgery, and Pharmacological Sciences, Executive Vice Chair, Program Director, Residency Training Program, Program Director, ASA Endorsed HELPS Simulation Program, Department of Anesthesiology, Perioperative and Pain Medicine, Icahn School of Medicine at Mount Sinai, New York, New York, USA

SATISH GOVINDARAJ, MD, FACS, FARS
Associate Professor, Departments of Otolaryngology–Head and Neck Surgery and Neurosurgery, Vice Chairman of Clinical Affairs, Department of Otolaryngology–Head and Neck Surgery, Icahn School of Medicine at Mount Sinai, New York, New York, USA

SAMUEL DeMARIA Jr, MD
Professor, Departments of Anesthesiology, Perioperative and Pain Medicine and Otolaryngology–Head and Neck Surgery, Director, Division of Liver Transplantation, Department of Anesthesiology, Perioperative and Pain Medicine, Icahn School of Medicine at Mount Sinai, New York, New York, USA

AUTHORS

BASEM B. ABDELMALAK, MD
Professor of Anesthesiology, Departments of General Anesthesiology and Outcomes Research, Anesthesiology Institute, Cleveland Clinic, Cleveland, Ohio, USA; President, Society for Head and Neck Anesthesia

CARLOS A. ARTIME, MD
Associate Professor and Clinical Executive Vice Chair, Department of Anesthesiology, McGovern Medical School, The University of Texas Health Science Center at Houston, Associate Operating Room Director, Memorial Hermann Hospital - Texas Medical Center, Houston, Texas, USA

GARRETT BURNETT, MD
Assistant Professor, Department of Anesthesiology, Perioperative and Pain Medicine, Icahn School of Medicine at Mount Sinai, New York, New York, USA

SAMUEL DeMARIA Jr, MD
Professor, Departments of Anesthesiology, Perioperative and Pain Medicine and Otolaryngology–Head and Neck Surgery, Director, Division of Liver Transplantation, Department of Anesthesiology, Perioperative and Pain Medicine, Icahn School of Medicine at Mount Sinai, New York, New York, USA

ELLEN S. DEUTSCH, MD, MS, FACS, FAAP, CPPS, FSSH
Adjunct Associate Professor, Anesthesiology and Critical Care, Senior Scientist, Department of Anesthesiology and Critical Care Medicine, University of Pennsylvania Perelman School of Medicine, Children's Hospital of Philadelphia, Philadelphia, Pennsylvania, USA

SHANE C. DICKERSON, MD
Assistant Clinical Professor of Anesthesiology, University of Southern California, Los Angeles, California, USA

DANIEL JOHN DOYLE, MD, PhD, DPhil
Department of General Anesthesiology, Cleveland Clinic Abu Dhabi, Abu Dhabi, United Arab Emirates; Professor of Anesthesiology, Cleveland Clinic Lerner College of Medicine, Cleveland, Ohio, USA

CARIN A. HAGBERG, MD
Chief Academic Officer, Division Head, Anesthesiology, Critical Care and Pain Medicine, Helen Shaffer Fly Distinguished Professor of Anesthesiology, Department of Anesthesiology and Perioperative Medicine, The University of Texas MD Anderson Cancer Center, Houston, Texas, USA

ANASTASIOS G. HANTZAKOS, MD, PhD, MHA, FEBORL
Clinical Assistant Professor of Otolaryngology, Cleveland Clinic Lerner College of Medicine, Cleveland, Ohio, USA; Department of Otolaryngology–Head and Neck Surgery, Cleveland Clinic Abu Dhabi, Abu Dhabi, United Arab Emirates

NARASIMHAN "SIM" JAGANNATHAN, MD, MBA
Professor of Anesthesiology, Northwestern University Feinberg School of Medicine, Associate Chair, Academic Affairs Director, Pediatric Anesthesia Research, Department of Pediatric Anesthesiology, Ann & Robert H. Lurie Children's Hospital of Chicago, Chicago, Illinois, USA

FREEDOM JOHNSON, MD, FACS
Department of Otolaryngology–Head and Neck Surgery, Director, Head and Neck Oncologic, Reconstructive and Cranial Base Surgery, Assistant Professor, Associate Residency Program Director, Case Western Reserve University School of Medicine, MetroHealth Medical Center, Cleveland, Ohio, USA

YURY KHELEMSKY, MD
Departments of Anesthesiology, Perioperative and Pain Medicine, and Neurology, Associate Professor, Icahn School of Medicine at Mount Sinai, New York, New York, USA

JOHN D. LANG Jr, MD
Professor, Department of Anesthesiology and Pain Medicine, University of Washington School of Medicine, Seattle, Washington, USA

ADAM I. LEVINE, MD
Professor, Departments of Anesthesiology, Perioperative and Pain Medicine, Otolaryngology–Head and Neck Surgery, and Pharmacological Sciences, Executive Vice Chair, Program Director, Residency Training Program, Program Director, ASA Endorsed HELPS Simulation Program, Department of Anesthesiology, Perioperative and Pain Medicine, Icahn School of Medicine at Mount Sinai, New York, New York, USA

ALDO V. LONDINO III, MD
Assistant Professor of Otolaryngology, The Mount Sinai Hospital, New York, New York, USA

JESSICA LOVICH-SAPOLA, MD, MBA, FASA
Associate Professor, Case Western Reserve University School of Medicine, President-Elect of the Medical Staff, Attending Anesthesiologist, Director of Anesthesia Quality, MetroHealth Medical Center, Member of the American Society of Anesthesiologists, Committee on Trauma and Emergency Preparedness, Cleveland, Ohio, USA

CHRISTINE L. MAI, MD, MS-HPEd
Assistant Professor, Department of Anesthesia, Critical Care and Pain Medicine, Massachusetts General Hospital, Boston, Massachusetts, USA

DAVID K. MADTES, MD
Associate Professor, Medicine Department, Division of Pulmonary and Critical Care Medicine, University of Washington School of Medicine, Seattle, WA, USA

ANUJ MALHOTRA, MD
Department of Anesthesiology, Perioperative and Pain Medicine, Assistant Professor, Icahn School of Medicine at Mount Sinai, New York, New York, USA

BRETT A. MILES, DDS, MD
Professor, Department of Otolaryngology and Head and Neck Surgery, Icahn School of Medicine at Mount Sinai, New York, New York, USA

BHARAT AKHANDA PANUGANTI, MD
Department of Surgery, Division of Otolaryngology–Head and Neck Surgery, University of California, San Diego, San Diego, California, USA

LEOPOLDO V. RODRIGUEZ, MD, FAAP, FASA
President-Elect, Society for Ambulatory Anesthesiology (SAMBA), Member, Committee on Ambulatory Surgical Care and Committee on Performance and Outcome Measures, American Society of Anesthesiologists, Medical Director, Surgery Center of Aventura, Aventura, Florida, USA; Assistant National Medical Director, Ambulatory Anesthesiology Division, Envision Physician Services, Plantation, Florida, USA

SOHAM ROY, MD, FACS, FAAP
Professor and Vice Chairman, Department of Otorhinolaryngology–Head and Neck Surgery, Chief of Pediatric Otolaryngology–Head and Neck Surgery, Director of Quality and Safety, Director of Undergraduate Medical Education, Assistant Dean, Admissions and Student Affairs, McGovern Medical School, The University of Texas Health Science Center at Houston, Children's Memorial Hermann Hospital, Houston, Texas, USA

ANJAN SHAH, MD
Assistant Professor of Anesthesiology, Department of Anesthesiology, Perioperative and Pain Medicine, Icahn School of Medicine at Mount Sinai, New York, New York, USA

RONAK SHAH, MD
Fellow in Simulation and Education, Department of Anesthesiology, Perioperative and Pain Medicine, Icahn School of Medicine at Mount Sinai, New York, New York, USA

MOURAD SHEHEBAR, MD
Department of Anesthesiology, Perioperative and Pain Medicine, Assistant Professor, Icahn School of Medicine at Mount Sinai, New York, New York, USA

CHARLES E. SMITH, MD
Attending Anesthesiologist and Director of Anesthesia Research, Department of Anesthesiology, Professor, Case Western Reserve University School of Medicine, MetroHealth Medical Center, Cleveland, Ohio, USA

JASPREET SOMAL, MBBS
Department of Anesthesiology and Critical Care, University of California, San Diego, San Diego, California, USA

TRACEY STRAKER, MD, MS, MPH, CBA, FASA
Professor, Department of Anesthesiology, Montefiore Medical Center, The University Hospital for Albert Einstein College of Medicine, Bronx, New York, USA; Adjunct Clinical Professor of Medicine, CUNY School of Medicine, New York, New York, USA

WENDY M. SUHRE, MD
Assistant Professor, Department of Anesthesiology and Pain Medicine, University of Washington School of Medicine, Seattle, Washington, USA

ANTHONY TANELLA, MD
Resident Physician, Department of Anesthesiology, Icahn School of Medicine at Mount Sinai, New York, New York, USA

PHILIP A. WEISSBROD, MD
Department of Surgery, Division of Otolaryngology–Head and Neck Surgery, University of California, San Diego, San Diego, California, USA

DOUGLAS M. WORRALL, MD
Resident Physician, Department of Otolaryngology–Head and Neck Surgery, Icahn School of Medicine at Mount Sinai, New York, New York, USA

Contents

Agreement between surgical and anesthesia teams regarding appropriate perioperative management strategies is vital to delivering safe and effective patient care. Perioperative guidelines serve as a valuable reference in optimizing patients for surgery. The article provides a broad set of guidelines related to cardiovascular evaluation, medication reconciliation, and preoperative fasting and includes a framework for the care of patients with comorbidities, such as coronary artery disease and obstructive sleep apnea.

Simulation-based education (SBE) has become pervasive in health care training and medical education, and is even more important in subspecialty training whereby providers such as otolaryngologists and anesthesiologists share overlapping patient concerns because of the proximity of the surgical airway. Both these subspecialties work in a fast-paced environment involving high-stakes situations and life-changing events that necessitate critical thinking and timely action, and have an exceedingly small bandwidth for error. Team training in the form of interprofessional education and learning involving surgeons, anesthesiologists, and nursing is critical for patient safety in the operating room in general, but more so in otolaryngology surgery.

Anesthesiologists and otolaryngologists share the airway in an elegant ballet that requires communication, collaboration, and mutual respect. This article addresses principles to prevent or manage challenging conditions such as airway fires, anatomically difficult airways, and post-tonsillectomy hemorrhage. Discussion includes rationales for the use of simulation and resilience engineering principles to achieve the safest patient care.

Blunt, penetrating trauma to the ear, nose, and throat, and related structures are striking. Injuries may range from simple soft tissue wounds to complex injuries of the face, neck, and brain. Proximity of the cervical spine and airway complicate anesthetic management. A multidisciplinary approach is required. Airway control has highest priority in initial care. Management of airway, breathing, and circulation need to be tailored to the patient. Decisions regarding airway management, ventilation strategies, monitoring, and fluid and blood administration should be based on the patient's condition, clinical setting, and the available personnel, expertise, and equipment.

Airway endoscopy (rigid and flexible bronchoscopy) is an important procedure that allows for visualization of the trachea and bronchi as well as treatment of a variety of airway disorders for diagnostic and therapeutic interventions. Excellent communication between the anesthesiologist and the endoscopist is required to ensure that adequate oxygenation and ventilation is maintained via the shared airway. Various anesthetic and airway management techniques can be used for airway management in pediatric foreign-body aspiration. This article highlights indications, techniques, and complications encountered during pediatric bronchoscopy, with particular focus on anesthetic management of the pediatric airway.

Via the emergence of new bronchoscopic technologies and techniques, there is enormous growth in the number of procedures being performed in nonoperating room settings. This, coupled with a greater focus from the Centers for Medicare and Medicaid Services for mandated anesthesiology oversight of procedural sedation for bronchoscopy by the pulmonologists has led to a more frequent working partnership between interventional pulmonologists and anesthesiologists. This article offers the interventional pulmonologist insight into how the anesthesiologist thinks and approaches anesthetic care delivery.

Regional anesthesia and acute pain management in otolaryngology uses multimodal techniques for perioperative pain control. Multiple methods for regional anesthesia and acute pain management are discussed, including indications and techniques for decreasing perioperative opioid requirements and enhancing recovery.

Anuj Malhotra, Mourad Shehebar, and Yury Khelemsky

The reasons for development of chronic pain are poorly understood. Chronic postoperative pain is linked to severe acute postoperative pain. Head and neck pain is often a complex phenomenon that requires meticulous diagnosis and treatment. Institution of early multimodal analgesic regimens by multidisciplinary teams may attenuate chronic pain formation and propagation in the otolaryngologic patient.

Douglas M. Worrall, Anthony Tanella, Samuel DeMaria Jr, and Brett A. Miles

Enhanced recovery protocols have been developed from gastrointestinal, colorectal, and thoracic surgery populations. The basic tenets of head and neck enhanced recovery are: a multidisciplinary team working around the patient, preoperative carbohydrate loading, multimodal analgesia, early mobilization and oral feeding, and frequent reassessment and auditing of protocols to improve patient outcomes. The implementation of enhanced recovery protocols across surgical populations appear to decrease length of stay, reduce cost, and improve patient satisfaction without sacrificing patient quality of care or changing readmission rates. This article examines evidence-based enhanced recovery interventions and tailors them to a major head and neck surgery population.

Carlos A. Artime, Soham Roy, and Carin A. Hagberg

Airway management is a cornerstone of anesthetic practice, and difficulty with airway management has potentially grave implications—failure to secure a patent airway can result in hypoxic brain injury or death in a matter of minutes. The difficult airway in otolaryngologic surgery requires careful planning and close communication between the anesthesiologist and ENT or head and neck surgeon. Knowledge of predictive factors and a detailed preoperative evaluation can be used to predict which airway strategies are likely to be successful and which are likely to fail.

Daniel John Doyle and Anastasios G. Hantzakos

Airway narrowing can be idiopathic or can occur as a result of airway tumors, hematomas, infections, and other pathologic conditions. Endoscopic management variously involves balloon dilatation, stent placement, laser vaporization of pathologic tissue, microdebridement, and other interventions, using either a rigid or a flexible bronchoscope. Jet ventilation is frequently used in such settings, especially when the presence of an endotracheal tube would interfere with the procedure. In desperate cases, extracorporeal membrane oxygenation may be used in managing the critical airway.

Head and neck surgical patients, at times, can represent a challenging population to manage in the intensive care unit postoperatively. Close interaction between the critical care and surgical teams, awareness of potential surgery-specific complications, and utilization of protocol-driven care can reduce risk of morbidity significantly in this population and enhance outcomes. Given the relative complexity of otolaryngologic surgery and the unique risk that head and neck pathologies can pose to patient airway, breathing, and circulation, these collective circumstances warrant detailed discussion in the interest of minimizing patient morbidity and mortality.

With today's technological advances in outpatient surgery, anesthetic technique does not differ significantly between inpatient and outpatient settings. It is important to decide which setting is most appropriate for the patient based on the surgeon's ability, the patient's comorbidities, the facility resources, and the staff who will provide care for the patient. Matching all of the above can lead to good outcomes, less complications, and a good patient experience.

OTOLARYNGOLOGIC CLINICS
OF NORTH AMERICA

FORTHCOMING ISSUES

February 2020
Cranial Nerve Stimulation in Otolaryngology
James G. Naples and Michael J. Ruckenstein, *Editors*

April 2020
Ethnically Sensitive Rhinoplasty
Lisa Ishii, Anthony Brissett and Kofi Boahene, *Editors*

June 2020
Sleep Apnea
Ofer Jacobowitz, Maria Suurna, *Editors*

RECENT ISSUES

October 2019
Pediatric Otolaryngology
Samantha Anne, Julina Ongkasuwan, *Editors*

August 2019
Advancements in Clinical Laryngology
Jonathan M. Bock, Chandra M. Ivey and Karen B. Zur, *Editors*

June 2019
Office-Based Surgery in Otolaryngology
Melissa A. Pynnonen and Cecelia E. Schmalbach, *Editors*

SERIES OF RELATED INTEREST

Facial Plastic Surgery Clinics
Available at: https://www.facialplastic.theclinics.com/

THE CLINICS ARE AVAILABLE ONLINE!
Access your subscription at:
www.theclinics.com

OTOLARYNGOLOGIC CLINICS
OF NORTH AMERICA

Foreword

Working Together from Both Sides of the Curtain

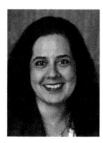

Sujana S. Chandrasekhar, MD, FACS, FAAOHNS
Consulting Editor

All surgeons and anesthesiologists partner with each other in order to provide high-quality operative care. In Otolaryngology, specifically, the communication between surgeon and anesthesiologist is intimate and can be very complicated. Guest editors Drs Adam Levine, Samuel DeMaria, and Satish Govindaraj have crafted this issue of *Otolaryngologic Clinics of North America* to address the very particular concerns that are raised when these 2 types of specialists are providing care to a single patient.

What are those concerns? While other types of cases involve a curtain separating surgeon and anesthesiologist, we often share the airway with each other, and that airway may look dramatically different from the beginning of a given case to the end. ENT procedures may involve acute airway compromise, such as in cases of peritonsillar abscess, epiglottitis, airway foreign body, or tumor- or trauma-related difficult airway. Conversely, Otolaryngology procedures themselves may risk acute airway compromise in a previously relatively normal condition, such as in the cases of pediatric and adult bronchoscopy or sleep endoscopy. There can be intubation concerns when the surgery is being performed for voice enhancement, such as direct laryngoscopy for vocal fold nodules or edema, or medialization laryngoplasty.

There are other areas of professional overlap. During sinus and anterior skull-base surgery there are concerns about blood pressure levels and bleeding that must be communicated before, during, and after the case. During ear and lateral skull-base surgery, the patient's head and airway are far from the anesthesiologist, who is stationed at the foot of the bed, and nonparalytic anesthesia must be maintained while avoiding even the slightest amount of patient movement. Surgical management of neck masses in adults and children can pose another set of challenges.

Most routine otolaryngology cases are ambulatory or same-day procedures. This means that while the correct depth of anesthesia is needed, the primary effects must be gone in a relatively short period of time so that the patient can go home.

Otolaryngol Clin N Am 52 (2019) xiii–xiv
https://doi.org/10.1016/j.otc.2019.09.007
0030-6665/19/© 2019 Published by Elsevier Inc.

For cases being performed in office procedure rooms, there are particular nuances that maximize care. In the case of patients who are sicker or who have more involved surgery that requires admission, our colleagues in Anesthesia can provide enhanced pain management and recovery.

"If we fail to prepare, we prepare to fail." This paraphrased quote from Benjamin Franklin highlights the importance of the opening articles in this issue of *Otolaryngologic Clinics of North America*. The surgeon understanding perioperative guidelines minimizes unnecessary delays or cancellations. Having access, particularly for trainees, to simulators and running virtual scenarios build knowledge as well as team collaboration. If each member of the team clearly communicates their concerns and the procedural goals, patient safety is markedly enhanced.

I commend Drs Levine, DeMaria, and Govindaraj on their selection of topics and authors. They have compiled a thorough, up-to-date issue of *Otolaryngologic Clinics of North America* on Anesthesia in Otolaryngology wherein the reader from each specialty can gain a better understanding of where we overlap and can work together to achieve the best patient outcomes.

Sujana S. Chandrasekhar, MD, FACS, FAAOHNS
Consulting Editor, Otolaryngologic Clinics of North America

Past President, American Academy of Otolaryngology-Head and Neck Surgery,
Secretary-Treasurer, American Otological Society
Partner, ENT & Allergy Associates, LLP
18 East 48th Street, 2nd Floor
New York, NY 10017, USA

Clinical Professor, Department of Otolaryngology-Head and Neck Surgery
Zucker School of Medicine at Hofstra-Northwell
Hempstead, NY, USA

Clinical Associate Professor
Department of Otolaryngology-Head and Neck Surgery
Icahn School of Medicine at Mount Sinai
New York, NY, USA

E-mail address:
ssc@nyotology.com

Preface

Anesthesiology and Otolaryngology: A Critical and Unique Collaboration of Specialist and Specialties

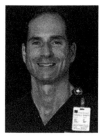 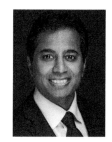 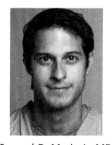

Adam I. Levine, MD   Satish Govindaraj, MD, FACS, FARS   Samuel DeMaria Jr, MD
Editors

The fields of anesthesiology and otolaryngology are forever linked due to the physical proximity and the sharing of one of the most critical anatomic structures, the airway. What started as informal discussions and an appreciation of the intimate connection of our mutual specialties among the 3 of us many years ago has evolved into a close professional collaboration and friendship. In 2013, those discussions culminated in creating one of the first textbooks of its kind, *Anesthesiology and Otolaryngology*,[1] a comprehensive text that brought together teams of anesthesiologists and otolaryngologists to discuss topics based on each other's point of view. The text fostered an appreciation of the intricacies involved in one another's specialty. In essence, putting into the printed word the same discussions and communications that should be taking place between anesthesiologists and otolaryngologist on a daily basis with respect to patient safety and care. This issue of *Otolaryngologic Clinics of North America* is in many ways an extension of this prior work, focusing on areas that are pertinent more to the anesthesiologist, but providing an otolaryngologist perspective in select areas, such as adult and pediatric bronchoscopy, where both specialties must work closely together where communication and team work are paramount.

The first 3 articles in this issue of *Otolaryngologic Clinics of North America* focus on key introductory topics in the field of anesthesia that serve as an overview for the otolaryngologist. Perioperative Guidelines, Simulation and Education, and Patient Safety are 3 areas that set a firm foundation to the reader before discussing more focused topics. The rest of the articles were chosen based on clinical situations where efficient and timely decisions need to be made between anesthesiologists and

Otolaryngol Clin N Am 52 (2019) xv–xvi
https://doi.org/10.1016/j.otc.2019.09.016
0030-6665/19/© 2019 Published by Elsevier Inc.

otolaryngologists, such as in head and neck trauma and adult and pediatric bronchoscopy. The management of the difficult airway and narrow airway is covered separately as each entity has unique aspects in their management and requires a refined collaboration between the anesthesiologist and otolaryngologist. The remaining articles in this issue cover acute and chronic pain management, enhanced recovery protocols after head and neck surgery, postoperative care, and last, anesthesia in the ambulatory and office setting.

The goal of this issue is to provide a comprehensive overview of the key issues in anesthesia as they relate to otolaryngology. Readers will have a concise presentation of each topic in a single source for future reference. It is our expectation that anesthesiologists as well as otolaryngologists will find the content of this issue a valuable adjunct in the perioperative management of the otolaryngology patient.

Adam I. Levine, MD
Department of Anesthesiology, Perioperative and Pain Management
One Gustave L. Levy Place, Box 1010
New York, NY 10029, USA

Satish Govindaraj, MD, FACS, FARS
Department of Otolaryngology–HNS
Mount Sinai Health System
234 East 85th Street, 4th Floor
New York, NY 10029, USA

Samuel DeMaria Jr, MD
Department of Anesthesiology, Perioperative and Pain Management
One Gustave L. Levy Place, Box 1010
New York, NY 10029, USA

E-mail addresses:
Adam.levine@mountsinai.org (A.I. Levine)
Satish.govindaraj@mountsinai.org (S. Govindaraj)
Samuel.demariajr@mountsinai.org (S. DeMaria)

REFERENCE

1. Levine AI, DeMaria S Jr, Schwartz A, et al. The comprehensive textbook of healthcare simulation. New York: Springer Science and Business Media; 2013.

Perioperative Guidelines in Anesthesia

Shane C. Dickerson, MD

KEYWORDS

- Cardiovascular assessment • Preoperative diagnostic studies
- Medication management • NPO guidelines • Percutaneous coronary intervention
- Obstructive sleep apnea

KEY POINTS

- Preoperative evaluation involves patient risk stratification and assessment of functional status. In those with questionable or indeterminate functional status, formal cardiac evaluation may be required.
- Routine laboratory panels, electrocardiograms, and chest radiographs are unnecessary in healthy, asymptomatic patients presenting for low-risk surgery.
- Perioperative medication management can be complicated and requires clear communication between practitioner and patient.
- Identification of at-risk patients and implementation of a multimodal prophylactic regimen aid in preventing perioperative nausea and vomiting.
- Patients presenting with coronary stents or permanent pacemakers and those with obstructive sleep apnea present a unique set of concerns to physicians.

INTRODUCTION

Optimal perioperative management of patients presenting for otolaryngologic surgery is multifaceted and requires an individualized approach to each patient. Evaluation and preparation prior to the day of surgery must include an assessment of cardiovascular status, sound medication reconciliation, and recognition of patient-specific concerns that may require additional planning in order to deliver safe care and minimize risk. Often, the indication for surgery is merely one of many medical issues encountered by practitioners when caring for patients. Focus on patients' complete medical profile must be maintained to facilitate desired surgical outcomes. To properly navigate complex medical issues and to ensure proper evidence-based practice, adherence to existing guidelines is key.

Disclosure Statement: None.
University of Southern California, 1450 San Pablo Street, Suite 3600, Los Angeles, CA 90033, USA
E-mail address: shane.dickerson@med.usc.edu

Otolaryngol Clin N Am 52 (2019) 981–993
https://doi.org/10.1016/j.otc.2019.08.001   oto.theclinics.com
0030-6665/19/© 2019 Elsevier Inc. All rights reserved.

PERIOPERATIVE ASSESSMENT

Safe delivery of both anesthetic and surgical care involves proper perioperative assessment of patient risk prior to surgery. The American Society of Anesthesiologists (ASA) scoring system provides a means by which patient risk can be stratified based on underlying comorbidities and surgical urgency. Originally developed for data standardization purposes and summarized in **Table 1**, the ASA scoring system is now ubiquitous in perioperative medicine and serves as an easily understood indicator of patient health across medical disciplines[1-3] (see **Table 1**).

In addition to the ASA scoring system, specific assessment of cardiac risk can be undertaken via utilization of several existing indices. The Revised Cardiac Risk Index was introduced more than 20 years ago and has become a trusted tool for providers to assess cardiac risk in a relatively facile manner. The index is composed of 5 patient-specific risk factors, which include history of congestive heart failure, coronary artery disease (CAD), cerebrovascular accident, insulin-dependent diabetes mellitus, and chronic kidney disease (creatinine >2). The final parameter takes the inherent risk of surgery into consideration by assigning a point to high-risk procedures, such as suprainguinal vascular, intraperitoneal, or intrathoracic surgery.[4] The percentage risks associated with each score are

- 0—class I risk, 0.4%
- 1—class II risk, 0.9%
- 2—class III risk, 6 .6%
- 3 to 0—class IV risk, 11%

Most head and neck surgeries are considered low risk. Increasing scores are associated with an increased risk of an adverse perioperative cardiac event.[5]

PREOPERATIVE DIAGNOSTIC STUDIES

Perioperative tests of cardiac function play an important role in proper optimization of patients prior to surgery. Overutilization of such tests places an undue economic burden on both the patient and health care system, and use of such tests must be undertaken with proper knowledge of the latest consensus guidelines. In some instances, a history and physical examination are the only assessments required prior to surgery. For example, everyday activities can be used as a surrogate for oxygen utilization and, in patients with adequate functional status undergoing low-risk surgery,

Table 1 American Society of Anesthesiologists physical status classification system	
Score	**Definition**
1	Healthy patient
2	Patient with mild systemic disease
3	Patient with severe systemic disease
4	Patient with severe disease that is a constant threat to life
5	Patient who is not expected to survive without surgery
6	A declared brain-dead patient
E	Indicates emergency surgery

Data from ASA physical status classification system. Committee of origin: standards and guidelines (approved by the ASA House of Delegates on October 15, 2014). Available at: https://www.asahq.org/standards-and-guidelines/asa-physical-status-classification-system. Accessed January 18, 2019.

no diagnostic studies or interventions are required prior to proceeding to the operating room. Metabolic equivalents help to quantify functional status, and patients who can carry out 4 or more metabolic equivalents are low risk for perioperative cardiac events[4,6] (**Table 2**).

Unfortunately, a significant number of patients present with diminished functional status, and, in some, assessment of functional status is impossible given underlying comorbidities. Under these circumstances, the algorithm outlined in **Fig. 1** provides a succinct pathway through which the need for cardiovascular testing can be determined.

Often patients receive routine laboratory studies in addition to an electrocardiogram (ECG) and/or chest x-ray (CXR) as part of a preoperative clearance. Emerging evidence suggests that these tests are unnecessary in asymptomatic individuals preparing for surgery. Per the ASA, routine ECG is unnecessary in most patients presenting for surgery unless clinical suspicion for cardiovascular disease exists. Although cardiovascular disease is more likely in the elderly population, extreme age alone is not an indication for an ECG in an elderly individual with good functional status.[7] The American Heart Association guidelines stipulate routine ECG is unnecessary in patients with underlying cardiovascular risk factors undergoing low risk surgery.[4] If, however, such a patient presents for intermediate-risk or high-risk surgery, an ECG should be considered.[8,9]

Routine CXR is recommended only in patients with underlying cardiopulmonary disease undergoing high risk surgery.[10] Risk factors, such as smoking and stable cardiopulmonary disease, should not be viewed as an impetus to obtain a CXR. The recommendation is supported by the limited utility of CXR to predict perioperative morbidity.[11]

Routine laboratory studies are not indicated in the absence of clinical suspicion for an abnormality that may alter patient management.[12] For example, an assessment of hematologic status is reasonable in patients with underlying anemia or liver disease because is a coagulation panel in a patient with a history of bleeding diathesis. In patients with kidney or liver disease, an electrolyte panel may be considered. Lastly, a urinalysis is unnecessary in many cases save for procedures involving the urinary tract or procedures involving the use of implants.[3,8]

MEDICATION MANAGEMENT

An important component of patient optimization prior to surgery entails proper medication reconciliation and a clear plan between practitioner and patient regarding any regimen changes in anticipation of surgery. In this instance, clear communication is vital as noncompliance or poor understanding can contribute to patient morbidity.

Table 2 Metabolic equivalents and examples	
Metabolic Equivalents	**Examples**
1	Basal metabolic rate at rest
<4	Slow dancing, golfing with cart, playing musical instrument
>4	Climbing 1 flight of stairs, walking up a hill, heavy house work

Data from Fleisher LA, Fleischmann KE, Uretsky BF, et al. 2014 ACC/AHA guideline on perioperative cardiovascular evaluation and management of patients undergoing noncardiac surgery. JACC 2014;64(22):e77-e137.

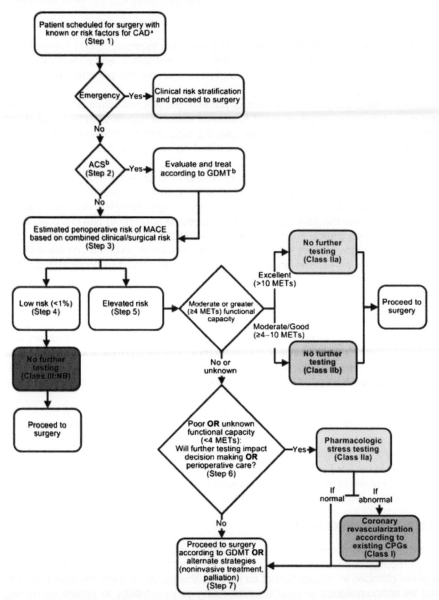

Fig. 1. Algorithm for preoperative cardiac assessment in patients with known/suspected CAD. In the setting of patients with known/suspected CAD, the acuity of the surgery combined with both surgery-specific and patient-specific risks must be collectively assessed to determine the need for further cardiac evaluation and potential intervention. The colors connote level of evidence, with green representing highest level of evidence and red the lowest. ACS, acute coronary syndrome; CPG, Clinical Practice Guidelines; GDMT, guideline-directed medical therapy; HF, heart failure; MACE, major adverse cardiovascular event; MET, metabolic equivalent; NB, no benefit; NSTEMI, non ST elevation myocardial infarction; STEMI, ST elevation myocardial infarction; UA, unstable angina; VHD, valvular heart disease. [a] See sections 2. 2, 2. 4, and 2.5 in the full-text CPG for recommendations for patients with symptomatic HF, VHD, or arrhythmias. [b] See UA/NSTEMI and STEMI CPGs (see **Table 2**). (*From* Fleisher LA, Fleischmann KE, Uretsky BF, et al. 2014 ACC/AHA guideline on perioperative cardiovascular evaluation and management of patients undergoing noncardiac surgery. JACC 2014;64(22):e77-e137; with permission.)

The following section provides recommendations for various classes of commonly used medications.

Cardiovascular Medications

β-Blocker therapy should be continued throughout the perioperative period.[13] Commencement of β-blocker therapy within 1 day of surgery should be avoided because doing so is associated with increased morbidity and mortality.[4,14] Because withdrawal from α_2-agonists, such as clonidine, is associated with rebound hypertension, these medications should be continued in the perioperative period.[13] Calcium channel blocker and statin therapy should not be interrupted in anticipation of surgery. Due to concerns for hypovolemia, hypotension, and electrolyte disturbances, diuretics should be discontinued on the day of surgery and resumed when deemed clinically appropriate. Although a consensus has yet to be reached, angiotensin-converting enzyme and angiotensin receptor blockers should generally be held 24 hours prior to surgery because failure to do so is associated with an increased risk of death and major vascular events.[13,15]

Pulmonary Medications and Glucocorticoids

β-Agonist, leukotriene, and glucocorticoid therapy should be continued in the perioperative period.[13] In patients requiring long-term glucocorticoid use, stress dosing remains controversial and is unnecessary for minor procedures. Evidence suggests that stress dosing confers minimal risks to patients, and, if a patient is at increased risk of adrenal crisis either due to hypothalamic-pituitary-adrenal axis suppression or the nature of an upcoming surgery, stress dosing is reasonable. An alternative involves refraining from empiric stress dosing and administering glucocorticoids if signs of adrenal insufficiency, such as refractory hypotension, manifest in the perioperative period.[16]

Antiplatelet and Antithrombotic Agents

Assessment of patient thromboembolic risk and perioperative bleeding is essential to making a sound decision regarding antithrombotic therapy in the perioperative period. In most instances, the indication for therapy stems from a history of atrial fibrillation, deep venous thrombosis/pulmonary embolism, or presence of a mechanical heart valve. The CHA_2-DS_2-VASc score for Stroke Risk Assessment in Atrial Fibrillation, the timing and frequency of deep venous thrombosis, and the type of valvular prosthesis are taken into consideration, respectively, when assessing thromboembolic risk in these scenarios.[17,18] The author strongly recommends obtaining the consultation of a cardiologist to help guide the perioperative anticoagulation strategy (ie, holding, bridging, and restarting) for patients with mechanical valves. In general, anticoagulation can be held safely in the perioperative period for those patients receiving it for stoke prophylaxis. Next, the surgery-specific bleeding risk is considered wherein tympanoplasty, diagnostic nasopharyngoscopy/laryngoscopy, fine-needle aspiration, and vocal cord injections are considered low bleeding risk procedures. All other otolaryngologic procedures confer a high bleeding risk (>1/5%).[19] Finally, the class of drug and its associated kinetic profile dictate discontinuation and reinstitution of therapy[18,20] (**Table 3**).

Situations may arise that require urgent discontinuation of antithrombotic therapy. Reversal of vitamin K antagonists, such as warfarin, entails the administration of either oral or intravenous vitamin K and potentially prothrombin complex concentrates or fresh frozen plasma depending on the timing and severity of bleeding.[18,21] Both unfractionated and low-molecular-weight heparin may be reversed with protamine

Table 3
Antithrombotic and antiplatelet medication overview

Medication	When to Stop Preoperatively	When to Restart Postoperatively
Aspirin	Continue, or 7–10 d	Continue, or 12–24 h
Clopidogrel, prasugrel, ticagrelor	5–7 d	24 h
Cilostazol	2 d	24 h
Ticlopidine	7–10 d	24 h
Warfarin	4–5 d	12–24 h
Unfractionated heparin	4–6 h (IV); 8–12 h (SQ)	12–24 h
Low-molecular-weight heparin	24 h	1–3 d
Fondaparinux	36–42 h	6–24 h
Dabigatran, rivaroxaban, apixaban,	1–3 d[a]	1–3 d[a]
Argatroban	4 h	1–3 d

[a] Assumes normal creatinine clearance and renal function. In patients with impaired renal function, a longer period of cessation may be necessary.

Adapted from Meyer A, Gross N, Teng M. AHNS series: do you know your guidelines? Perioperative antithrombotic management in head and neck surgery. Head & Neck 1028;40:182-191; with permission.

sulfate.[21] Idarucizumab is a Food and Drug Administration–approved antidote for the direct thrombin inhibitor dabigatran.[22] Recently, Andexanet alfa was approved in the United States as a reversal agent for the factor Xa inhibitors apixaban and rivaroxaban.[23]

Diabetic Agents

The appropriate timing of antihyperglycemic therapy is essential to proper glucose management in the perioperative period, but effective glucose management can prove difficult secondary to the stress response elicited by surgical intervention. On the day prior to surgery, patients can abide by their normal regimens except in those who administer basal insulin (glargine or detemir) or intermediate-acting insulin (isophane insulin or 70/30 insulin) at nighttime. The doses of each should be reduced to 80% of the usual dose on the evening preceding surgery.[24]

Oral antihyperglycemics, noninsulin injectables, and short-acting insulin (lispro or aspart) should all be held on the day of surgery. The morning dose of basal insulin should be reduced by 20%, and intermediate-acting insulin requires a 50% reduction if blood glucose levels are above 120 mg/dL.[24]

Perioperatively, glucose levels should be measured prior to surgery and at least every 2 hours thereafter. Treatment of hyperglycemia with either subcutaneous or intravenous insulin is recommended for levels above 180 mg/dL. If hypoglycemia is encountered (glucose <70 mg/dL), a dextrose-containing solution should be administered with point-of-care glucose testing every 15 minutes until patients are normoglycemic. The basal bolus approach, which includes both sliding scale and basal insulin, is recommended in the postoperative period because sole reliance on the former can result in undesired glucose fluctuations.[24]

Insulin pumps may be continued intraoperatively provided the pump's location does not interfere with the surgical field. The pump's basal rate is maintained, and hourly glucose checks are recommended. The pump is turned off if serum glucose dips below 110 mg/dL, and physician-administered bolus doses are used to correct hyperglycemia (glucose >180 mg/dL). If the pump needs to be inactivated perioperatively, an insulin infusion set to the pump's basal rate should be instituted. It is recommended that patients manage their pumps independently once able to do so from a cognitive standpoint.[25]

FASTING, ASPIRATION PROPHYLAXIS, AND THE PREVENTION OF POSTOPERATIVE NAUSEA AND VOMITING

Adherence to perioperative fasting guidelines is an important factor in the prevention of pulmonary aspiration and its associated sequelae. Clear liquids, which include water, clear juices devoid of pulp, and plain coffee and tea, may be ingested up to 2 hours before a scheduled procedure. Breast milk must be held for 4 hours prior to a procedure, and 6 hours is required for nonhuman milk and infant formula. The required fasting period for meals involves assessment of the patient's current gastroenterological status as well as the type and size of meal. In general, 6 hours of fasting after meals is adequate. If a patient presents with risk factors consistent with delayed gastric emptying or if the meal is particularly large or high in fat, however, 8 hours of fasting is recommended.[26]

Nonparticulate antacids, gastric stimulants, H_2-receptor antihistamines, and proton pump inhibitors may be administered to patients at increased risk of pulmonary aspiration. Preoperative anticholinergics, however, should not be used in the same fashion.[26] In patients with esophageal pathology, such as a blind esophageal pouch or diverticula, pouch emptying and placement of an orogastric tube are recommended, respectively, prior to induction of anesthesia. An airway assessment is integral to the prevention of aspiration in those presenting with gastric distention. If difficult mask ventilation or laryngoscopy is anticipated, an awake intubation should be performed. In patients with reassuring airways, a nasogastric tube under suction should be utilized in individuals with moderate to severe gastric distention prior to a rapid sequence induction. Mild gastric distention requires a rapid sequence induction absent preemptive nasogastric tube placement.[27] Evidence on the use of routine cricoid pressure under these circumstances remains equivocal.[28]

Identification of patients at increased risk of postoperative nausea and vomiting (PONV) is the initial step in developing a sound prophylactic plan. Individual risk factors include female gender, history of PONV or motion sickness, nonsmoking status, and younger age. Procedure-specific risk factors include volatile anesthetic and nitrous oxide use and postoperative opioid use. Preferential use of regional or local anesthetic techniques should be used in high-risk patients when possible. Combination prophylactic antiemetic therapy is recommended, especially in moderate-risk to high-risk individuals. Staples of therapy include corticosteroids, 5HT-3 antagonists, neurokinin-1 antagonists, phenothiazines, antihistamines, and anticholinergics. In addition, adequate hydration has been demonstrated to decrease the risk of developing PONV.[29] Simplified PONV prophylactic and treatment algorithms are recommended because overly complex rubrics lead to poor application and execution.[30]

PATIENT-SPECIFIC CONCERNS
Prior Percutaneous Coronary Intervention

Timing is key to preventing untoward thrombotic events in individuals who have undergone recent percutaneous coronary intervention (PCI). There are generally 3 approaches to revascularization in those presenting with either stable ischemic heart disease (SIHD) or acute coronary syndrome (ACS): balloon angioplasty, bare metal stenting (BMS), or placement of a drug-eluting stent (DES). The appropriate timing for planning elective surgery after each intervention is outlined in **Table 4**. Patients

Table 4
Timing of elective noncardiac surgery after percutaneous coronary intervention

Intervention Type	Appropriate Timing of Elective Surgery
Balloon angioplasty	>14 d
BMS	>30 d
DES	>6 mo

Data from Fleisher LA, Fleischmann KE, Uretsky BF, et al. 2014 ACC/AHA guideline on perioperative cardiovascular evaluation and management of patients undergoing noncardiac surgery. JACC 2014;64(22):e77-e137 and Levine GN, Bates ER, Bittl JA, et al. 2016 ACC/AHA guideline focused update on duration of dual antiplatelet therapy in patients with coronary artery disease. JACC 2016;68(10):1082-1115.

who present in ACS with resultant PCI should be maintained on dual antiplatelet therapy (DAPT) for at least 12 months regardless of intervention type. DAPT typically consists of low-dose aspirin (81 mg) and a $P2Y_{12}$ inhibitor, such as clopidogrel. Recommendations differ in the setting of SIHD in which therapy should continue for a minimum of 14 days for balloon angioplasty, 1 month after BMS, and 6 months after DES.[4,31,32] Scenarios arise wherein the risk of delaying surgery in patients with recent PCI is significant, such as in the setting of malignancy. Under these circumstances, proceeding to surgery 3 months after DES placement can be considered.[31] Recent evidence suggests, however, that patients are increased risk of major adverse cardiac events (MACEs) when undergoing surgery within 180 days of DES placement, particularly in the first month postprocedure.[33,34] Aspirin therapy should be continued in the perioperative period for all ear, nose, and throat surgeries with the exception of those also involving surgeries conferring high bleeding risk, such as intracranial, intraspinal or intraocular surgery. Perioperative continuation and postsurgical resumption of $P2Y_{12}$ therapy should be determined by a team-based assessment of bleeding versus thrombotic risk.[31]

Permanent Pacemakers and Automated Internal Cardioverter-Defibrillators

The proper management of patients with implanted antiarrhythmic devices begins with a thorough history to ascertain a patient's device dependence as well as its type and function. Patients frequently present with a manufacturer information card detailing salient information. Preoperative interrogation is required if more than 6 months has elapsed since the most recent interrogation of an automated internal cardioverter-defibrillator (AICD) or 12 months for a permanent pacemaker (PPM). Intraoperatively, electrocautery and radiofrequency can result in malfunction. The use of bipolar electrocautery and ultrasonic scalpel is preferred to monopolar electrocautery. If monopolar electrocautery is necessary, the receiving plate should be positioned in a manner that prevents the flow of current in the vicinity of the PPM/AICD generator and leads.[35] The likelihood of electromagnetic interference is greatest when the source is within 15 cm (6 in) of the generator.[36] In most instances, a magnet placed at the generator site will inactivate cardioverter-defibrillator function or result in asynchronous pacing with AICDs and PPMs, respectively, but the response is variable. Magnet placement is recommended in surgeries taking place above the umbilicus, and magnets should be available in all cases involving patients with PPM/AICD.[36] The capability to pace/defibrillate independent of indwelling mechanism should always be available and can be accomplished via the use of transcutaneous pacing pads.[35] The pads should remain in place during the immediate postoperative period, and postoperative apparatus interrogation is advised if suspicion for device malfunction is high (eg, inappropriate discharge) or if proper interrogation was not obtained preoperatively in the setting of emergent surgery.[35,37]

Obstructive Sleep Apnea

Screening for the presence of obstructive sleep apnea (OSA) may be accomplished via the STOP-Bang scoring system[38] (**Table 5**). If suspicion is high and time permits, a sleep study may be obtained, and preoperative optimization, including but not limited to continuous positive airway pressure (CPAP)/noninvasive positive pressure ventilation (NIPPV), mandibular devices, and weight loss is recommended.[39] The probability of patients with OSA presenting with difficult airways is greater than in the general population, and appropriate preparation should be made when managing these patients.[40] A preference for regional and opioid-sparing techniques should be utilized when clinically feasible.[39,40] In addition, deep sedation is discouraged in favor of a secure airway in patients with OSA, and extubation should be carried out when patients are fully awake.[39] If a patient is admitted to the hospital after surgery, continuous pulse oximetry is recommended. Non-narcotic adjuncts are recommended as a mainstay of postoperative pain management to decrease reliance on opioids. If patient-controlled analgesia is required, continuous basal infusions are highly discouraged.[39] Additionally, patients should be encouraged to bring their home CPAP/NIPPV devices because doing so increases compliance rates in the postoperative period.[39] When choosing between inpatient and ambulatory settings for cases, the type of surgery, anesthetic required, need for postoperative opioids, and capacity of outpatient facility to adequately monitor and treat patients with OSA must be considered. In cases of same day surgery, observation of patients breathing room air while sleeping in the absence of significant oxygen desaturation serves as a benchmark required for safe discharge.[39]

Pregnancy

On occasion pregnant patients require urgent head and neck surgery. Specific concerns for both mother and fetus arise when caring for these patients. Purely elective surgery should be postponed until after delivery, and, if surgery is to be performed during pregnancy, doing so in the second trimester is recommended. The facility accommodating surgery under these circumstances should house obstetric, neonatal, and pediatric staff. Additionally, fetal heart rate (FHR) monitoring should be immediately available. In cases of a previable fetus, ascertaining FHR before and after surgery is

Table 5 STOP-Bang scoring system	
Parameter	**Score**
Snoring	1
Tiredness	1
Observed snoring	1
High blood pressure	1
Body mass index >35 kg/m^2	1
Age over 50	1
Neck circumference >40 cm	1
Male gender	1

Scores $\geq$3 are highly sensitive for the presence of OSA.
Data from Chung F, Subramanyam, Liao P, et al. High STOP-Bang score indicates a high probability of obstructive sleep apnea. BJA 2012;108(5):768-775.

satisfactory. Both contraction and FHR monitoring are required before and after surgery with a viable fetus. Continuous intraoperative fetal monitoring may be considered if the fetus is viable, obstetric surgical staff are available to intervene, the surgery is conducive to a potential emergent delivery, and informed consent for cesarean section has been obtained. The preceding provides a framework for care of a parturient presenting for surgery; however, specific planning should be carried out on a case-by-case basis with input from surgical, obstetric, and anesthesia staff.[41]

Ex-premature Infant

Compared with infants born at term, the ex-premature infant (<37 weeks' gestation) presenting for surgery is at increased risk of several perioperative complications, including postoperative apnea and retinopathy of prematurity (ROP). Increasing postconception age (PCA) is negatively correlated with the incidence of postoperative apnea and serves as the strongest predictor of risk, which is greatest in infants less than 44 weeks PCA.[42] Additional risk factors include anemia and prior history of apnea whereas a decreased risk is observed in infants who are small-for-gestational age.[43] Preventative measures include the administration of caffeine and theophylline. Close postoperative monitoring is recommended for full-term infants less than 44 weeks PCA and preterm infants less than 60 weeks PCA presenting for surgery.[42,43] A minimum of 12 consecutive hours free of apneic events should be observed in each prior to discharge.[43]

ROP is characterized by abnormal eye vessel growth that may progress to retinal detachment and ultimately blindness. Prematurity, low birthweight, mechanical ventilation, and high inspired oxygen tension are all risk factors for the development of ROP.[44] In high-risk infants, supplemental oxygen should be limited as much as possible, especially in individuals less than 44 weeks PCA.[44] Increased oxygen tension poses fewer risks in infants greater than 44 weeks PCA and in those with existing prethreshold ROP.[44]

SUMMARY

Preparing patients for upcoming surgical procedures can be arduous owing to the nature of an upcoming procedure, the complex medical history of the patient, or both. Often, patients present with concomitant comorbidities and complex medication regimens, the management of which poses many potential issues to practitioners. Unfortunately, surgery does not occur in a vacuum, and a plan integrating a patient's history and surgery-specific concerns must be formulated. Adherence to evidenced-based practice is essential to accomplishing this goal, and perioperative guidelines serve as a template through which an objective, concise care plan can be used to keep patients safe and increase the odds of a seamless recovery.

REFERENCES

1. Saklad M. Grading patients for surgical procedures. Anesthesiology 1941;2: 281–4.
2. Owens WD, Felts JA, Spitznagel EL. ASA physical status classifications: a study of consistency of ratings. Anesthesiology 1978;49:239–43.
3. ASA physical status classification system. Committee of origin: standards and guidelines (approved by the ASA House of Delegates on October 15, 2014). Available at: https://www.asahq.org/standards-and-guidelines/asa-physical-status-classification-system. Accessed January 18, 2019.
4. Fleisher LA, Fleischmann KE, Uretsky BF, et al. 2014 ACC/AHA guideline on perioperative cardiovascular evaluation and management of patients undergoing noncardiac surgery. J Am Coll Cardiol 2014;64(22):e77–137.

5. Lee TH, Marcantonio ER, Mangione CM, et al. Derivation and prospective validation of a simple index for prediction of cardiac risk of major noncardiac surgery. Circulation 1999;100:1043–9.

6. Reilly DF, McNeely MJ, Doerner D, et al. Self-reported exercise tolerance and the risk of serious perioperative complications. Arch Intern Med 1999;159:2185–92.

7. Apfelbaum JL, Connis RT, Nickinovich DG. Practice advisory for preanesthesia evaluation. An updated report by the American Society of Anesthesiologists task force on preanesthesia evaluation. Anesthesiology 2012;116(3):1–17.

8. Smetana GW. Preoperative medical evaluation of the adult healthy patient. In: Post TW, editor. UpToDate. Waltham (MA): UpToDate. Available at: https://www.uptodate.com/contents/preoperative-medical-evaluation-of-the-healthy-adult-patient?search=preoperative%20medical%20evaluation&source=search_result&selectedTitle=2~150&usage_type=default&display_rank=213. Accessed January 18, 2019.

9. Association of Anaesthetists of Great Britain and Ireland. AAGBI safety guideline. Pre-operative assessment and patient preparation. 2010. Available at: http://www.aagbi.org/sites/default/files/preop2010.pdf. Accessed January 18, 2019.

10. Smetana GW, Lawrence VA, Cornell JE. Preoperative pulmonary risk stratification for noncardiothoracic surgery: systematic review for the American College of Physicians. Ann Intern Med 2006;144(8):581–95.

11. Garcia-Miguel FJ, Seerano-Aguilar PG, Lopez-Bastida J. Preoperative assessment. Lancet 2003;362(9397):1749–57.

12. Smetana GW, Macpherson DS. The case against routine preoperative laboratory testing. Med Clin North Am 2003;87(1):7–40.

13. Muluk VM, Cohn SL, Whinney C. Perioperative medication management. In: Post TW, editor. UptoDate. Waltham (MA). Available at: https://www.uptodate.com/contents/perioperative-medication-management?search=perioperative%20medication%20management&source=search_result&selectedTitle=1~68&usage_type=default&display_rank=1. Accessed January 19, 2019.

14. Wijeysundera DN, Duncan D, Nkonde-Price C, et al. Perioperative beta blockade in noncardiac surgery: a systematic review for the 2014 ACC/AHA guideline on perioperative cardiovascular evaluation and management of patients undergoing noncardiac surgery: a report of the American College of Cardiology/American Heart Association Task Force on practice guidelines. J Am Coll Cardiol 2014; 22(9):2406–25.

15. Roshanov PS, Rochwerg B, Patel A, et al. Withholding versus continuing angiotensin-converting enzyme inhibitors or angiotensin II receptor blockers before noncardiac surgery. An analysis of the vascular events in noncardiac surgery patients cohort evaluation prospective cohort. Anesthesiology 2017;126:16–27.

16. Liu MM, Reidy AB, Saatee S, et al. Perioperative steroid management: approaches based on current evidence. Anesthesiology 2017;127:166–72.

17. January CT, Wann LS, Stevenson WG, et al. 2014 AHA/ACC/HRS guideline for the management of patients with atrial fibrillation. J Am Coll Cardiol 2014;64(21):e1–76.

18. Douketis JD. Perioperative management of patients receiving anticoagulants. In: Post TW, editor. UpToDate. Waltham (MA): UpToDate. Available at: https://www.uptodate.com/contents/perioperative-management-of-patients-receiving-anticoagulants?search=perioperative%20management%20of%20patients%20receiving%20anticoagulants&source=search_result&selectedTitle=1~150&usage_type=default&display_rank=1. Accessed January 21, 2019.

19. Hsueh WD, Hwang PH, Abuzeid WM. Perioperative management of antithrombotic therapy in common otolaryngologic surgical procedures: state of the art review. Otolaryngol Head Neck Surg 2015;153(4):493–503.
20. Meyer A, Gross N, Teng M. AHNS series: do you know your guidelines? Perioperative antithrombotic management in head and neck surgery. Head Neck 2018; 40:182–91.
21. Thomas S, Makris M. The reversal of anticoagulation in clinical practice. Clin Med 2018;18(4):314–9.
22. Pollack CV, Reilly PA, Eikelboom J, et al. Idarucizumab for dabigatran reversal. N Engl J Med 2015;373:511–20.
23. Heo YA. Adnexanet alpha: first global approval. Drugs 2018;78(1):1049–55.
24. Duggan EW, Klopman MA, Berry AJ, et al. The Emory University perioperative algorithm for the management of hyperglycemia and diabetes in non-cardiac surgery patients. Curr Diab Rep 2016;16:34.
25. Duggan EW, Carlson K, Umpierrez GE. Perioperative hyperglycemia management. Anesthesiology 2017;126(3):547–60.
26. American Society of Anesthesiologists Task Force on preoperative fasting and the use of pharmacologic agents to reduce the risk of pulmonary aspiration. Practice guidelines for preoperative fasting and the use of pharmacologic agents to reduce the risk of pulmonary aspiration: application to healthy patients undergoing elective procedures. Anesthesiology 2017;126:376–93.
27. Salem MR, Khorasani A, Saatee S, et al. Gastric tubes and airway management in patients at risk of aspiration: history, current concepts, and proposal of an algorithm. Anesth Analg 2014;118:569–79.
28. Algie CM, Mahar RK, Tan HB, et al. Effectiveness and risks of cricoid pressure during rapid sequence induction for endotracheal intubation. Cochrane Database Syst Rev 2015;(11):CD011656.
29. Gan TJ, Diemunsch P, Habib AS, et al. Consensus guidelines for the management of postoperative nausea and vomiting. Anesth Analg 2014;118:85–113.
30. Dewinter G, Staelens W, Veef E, et al. Simplified algorithm for the prevention of postoperative nausea and vomiting: a before-and-after study. Br J Anaesth 2018;120:9–13.
31. Levine GN, Bates ER, Bittl JA, et al. 2016 ACC/AHA guideline focused update on duration of dual antiplatelet therapy in patients with coronary artery disease. J Am Coll Cardiol 2016;68(10):1082–115.
32. Kristensen SD, Knuuti J, Saraste A, et al. 2014 ESC/ESA guidelines on non-cardiac surgery: cardiovascular assessment and management. Eur Heart J 2014;35:2383–431.
33. Smith BB, Warner MA, Warner NS, et al. Cardiac risk of noncardiac surgery after percutaneous coronary intervention with second-generation drug-eluting stents. Anesth Analg 2018. https://doi.org/10.1213/ANE.0000000000003408.
34. Egholm G, Kristensen SD, Thim T, et al. Risk associated with surgery within 12 months after coronary drug-eluting stent implantation. J Am Coll Cardiol 2016;68(24):2622–32.
35. American Society of Anesthesiologists Task Force on perioperative management of patients with cardiac implantable electronic devices. Practice advisory for the perioperative management of patients with cardiac implantable electronic devices: pacemakers and implantable cardioverter-defibrillators. Anesthesiology 2011;114:247–61.

36. Neelankavil JP, Thompson A, Mahajan A. Managing cardiovascular implantable electronic devices (CIEDs) during perioperative care. APSF Newsletter 2013; 28(2):29, 32–5.
37. Schulman PM. Perioperative management of patients with a pacemaker or implantable cardioverter-defibrillator. In: Post TW, editor. UpToDate. Waltham (MA): UpToDate. Available at: https://www.uptodate.com/contents/perioperative-management-of-patients-with-a-pacemaker-or-implantable-cardioverter-defibrillator?search=Perioperative%20management%20of%20patients%20with%20a%20pacemaker&source=search_result&selectedTitle=1~150&usage_type=default&display_rank=1. Accessed February 2, 2019.
38. Chung F, Subramanyam R, Liao P, et al. High STOP-bang score indicates a high probability of obstructive sleep apnea. Br J Anaesth 2012;108(5):768–75.
39. American Society of Anesthesiologists Task Force on perioperative management of obstructive sleep apnea. Practice guidelines for the perioperative management of patients with obstructive sleep apnea. Anesthesiology 2014;120:268–86.
40. Memtsoudis SG, Cozowicz C, Nagappa M, et al. Society of anesthesia and sleep medicine guideline on intraoperative management of adult patients with obstructive sleep apnea. Anesth Analg 2018;127:967–87.
41. Committee Opinion No. 696 American College of Obstetricians and Gynecologists. Nonobstetric surgery during pregnancy. Obstet Gynecol 2017;129:777–8.
42. Heitmiller ES, Koka R. Chapter 57: safety and outcome in pediatric anesthesia. In: Davis PJ, Cladis FP, editors. Smith's anesthesia for infants and children. 9th edition. Philadelphia: Elsevier; 2017. p. 1327–8.
43. Ghazal EA, Vadi MG, Mason LJ, et al. Chapter 4: preoperative evaluation, premedication, and induction of anesthesia. In: Cote CJ, Lerman J, Anderson BJ, editors. Cote and Lerman's a practice of anesthesia for infants and children. 6th edition. Philadelphia: Elsevier; 2019. p. 64–5.
44. Ricketts K, Valley RD, Bailey AG, et al. Chapter 34: anesthesia for ophthalmic surgery. In: Davis PJ, Cladis FP, editors. Smith's anesthesia for infants and children. 9th edition. Philadelphia: Elsevier; 2017. p. 905–7.

Simulation-Based Education and Team Training

Anjan Shah, MD[a],*, Christine L. Mai, MD, MS-HPEd[b], Ronak Shah, MD[a],
Adam I. Levine, MD[a]

KEYWORDS

- Otolaryngology anesthesia • ENT anesthesia • Simulation education
- Crisis resource management • Interprofessional education
- Interprofessional learning • Patient safety

KEY POINTS

- Simulation-based education provides experiential learning opportunities that can help facilitate interprofessional training experiences for otolaryngologists and anesthesiologists.
- Interprofessional learning involving surgeons, anesthesiologists, and nursing is critical for patient safety in the operating room in general, but more so in otolaryngology surgery.
- Interprofessional education via multidisciplinary team simulations can help uncover latent errors in a medical system and improve patient safety.

INTRODUCTION

The medical profession has changed radically over the years, with growing opportunities and incentives for health care providers to become subspecialized within internal medicine, surgery, anesthesiology, and radiology, to name a few. Although subspecialization results in health care providers who are proficient and masters within their niche, it detracts from providing holistic care to the patient, as the importance of understanding the pathophysiology, and medical or technical issues outside of a particular subspecialty, may not be as evident to the provider. With the advancement in technology over the years and the increasing surgical and technical complexity of cases, surgical subspecialization has had direct implications within anesthesiology. Specifically, otolaryngology deals with a unique set of challenges that demand high-quality education and training among and between

Disclosure Statement: The authors have nothing to disclose.
[a] Department of Anesthesiology, Perioperative and Pain Medicine, Icahn School of Medicine at Mount Sinai, 1 Gustave L. Levy Place, Klingenstein Clinical Center 8th Floor, PO Box 1010, New York, NY 10029, USA; [b] Department of Anesthesia, Critical Care and Pain Medicine, Massachusetts General Hospital, 55 Fruit Street, Boston, MA 02114, USA
* Corresponding author.
E-mail address: anjan.shah@mountsinai.org

otolaryngologists, anesthesiologists, and nursing colleagues to ensure and enhance patient safety. Both otolaryngologists and anesthesiologists work in a fast-paced environment filled with high-stakes situations and life-changing events that necessitate critical thinking and timely action, and have an exceedingly small bandwidth for error. To tackle these issues of patient safety in rare and critical events, mannequin-based simulation was pioneered concurrently in the anesthesia departments at Stanford University and the University of Florida to teach concepts of crisis resource management. Since the advent and adaptation of simulation within health care, simulation-based education has had a widespread influence over medical education and training.

Traditionally, residency training emphasized basic science knowledge whereby the old adage of "see one, do one, teach one" was based on an apprenticeship model.[1] Because of the limitations on duty hours, variable learning opportunities, restrictions present in health care, and mounting pressure for patient safety, traditional teaching methods were supplemented with the growing use of simulation. Since the 1980s, simulation-based education offered an experiential learning paradigm for training and assessment, with opportunities to improve medical knowledge, communication, and technical and decision-making skills for common as well as rare events. This paradigm shift to an outcomes-based education model has led to a change from strictly using summative assessment (assessment *of* learning) to employing formative assessment (assessment *for* learning) to encourage learners to reflect on their own learning experiences. Today, simulation has become pervasive and is incorporated into every level of medical education from nursing and medical school education, to residency and fellowship training, specialty board certification, continuing medical education, and for health care providers seeking re-entry into the medical field. Currently, simulation use in residency training is largely in silo and isolated to a specific specialty within medicine, resulting in gaps in interprofessional education (IPE). Promotion of simulation in the form of augmented reality and virtual reality may enhance interprofessional learning (IPL) and interdisciplinary team training, and improve patient safety. This article defines the difference between simulation and a simulator, reviews the history of simulation with contributions from anesthesiology and crew resource management from aviation, and discusses the application of simulation for interdisciplinary team training in the operating room. It concludes with examples of institutions that have incorporated simulation programs to train otolaryngologists and anesthesiologists to work together as an effective team.

DEFINING SIMULATORS AND SIMULATION

To begin with, it is important to understand the distinction between a simulator and a simulation, even though these terms are often used interchangeably. A simulator refers to a physical piece of equipment/device, or a representation of a task that is to be replicated. For example, a partial task trainer is a mannequin or device designed to allow participants to practice a clinical skill or task. Many are simple devices designed for learning or practicing specific procedures (eg, airway head for mask ventilation and laryngoscopy). Others are more sophisticated devices coupled with computer and robotic interface, which can enhance the physical and virtual aspects of the simulator for practicing more advanced skills (eg, bronchoscopy). A simulation or simulated environment makes use of simulators to imitate a particular task or clinical scenario in a controlled environment. The creation of a safe space to allow students and trainees to learn without causing harm to oneself or patients is paramount in the development of the simulation environment. The degree of fidelity of the environment (level of realism) can vary depending on the resources available, and the level of fidelity is often dictated by the particular teaching objective.

HISTORY OF SIMULATION AND INCORPORATION WITHIN HEALTH CARE/MEDICAL EDUCATION

Simulation in its primitive form has been around for centuries, with the military being one of the first fields to use it in the sixth century by developing the game of chess. Although technology-based simulation in aviation first began with the "blue box" flight trainer created by Edwin Link in 1929, it did not gain traction by the army until the mid-to-late 1930s after several fatal aviation accidents made it evident that repetitive pre-flight practice in a safe environment was necessary for the safety of onboard personnel.[2] Over the years, with the advent of computer technology, flight simulators became more advanced and popularized.

Unlike the aviation industry and the military, medicine was slower to adopt simulation into its education repertoire. Anesthesiology in particular has been the forerunner of simulation innovation in health care. An early innovator, Asmund Laerdal, in conjunction with Bjorn Lind and other anesthesiologists in Norway, created Resusci-Anne (Laerdal, Stavanger, Norway) in the early 1960s. This mannequin was a part-task trainer with an airway that could be manipulated to cause an obstruction that was initially designed to train mouth-to-mouth ventilation.[3,4] This model was further adapted to include a spring in the chest to allow for cardiac compressions, which led to widespread use in cardiopulmonary resuscitation training.[3,4] Around the same time in 1963 to 1964, Stephen Abrahamson and Howard Barrows recognized limitations in the traditional methodology of bedside teaching arising from the unreliable and inconsistent nature of various clinical conditions reported by the patients. They went on to describe the "Programmed Patient," actors who were designated as simulated patients and used to portray various clinical presentations for students to learn from.[2,5] This concept did not gain initial acceptance in the 1960s because of the expense at the time and belief that its utility was "unscientific."[2] Over time, the terminology changed to "standardized patient" in testing situations. Today, standardized patients are widely used in simulation education.

Abrahamson went on to build SimOne in the late 1960s in conjunction with Aerojet General Corporation. Equipped with blinking eyes, reactive pupils, chest wall movement with respiration, airway manipulation, responsiveness to a handful of drugs, and a palpable heartbeat associated with a blood pressure reading, it was the first computer-driven mannequin simulator designed to train anesthesiology trainees.[2–4] Only one unit was built; however, it was not accepted because of the enormous expense for the computing technology at the time. Furthermore, the apprentice-based model of medical education training at the time precluded it from commercialization. Advances in mathematics and computer technology led to the ability to create human physiologic modeling that revolutionized the modernized patient simulators. Both led by convictions to enhance patient safety under anesthesia, 2 teams simultaneously developed high-fidelity patient simulators: David Gaba from Stanford University created the Comprehensive Anesthesia Simulation Environment (CASE 1.2), and Michael Good and a multidisciplinary team at the University of Florida, Gainesville developed the Gainesville Anesthesia Simulator.[3] Both of these original companies and designs have been modified as newer technology has emerged, and now exist in medical education. Today, human patient simulators (HPS), such as the Laerdal SimMan and SimBaby (Laerdal Medical, Stavanger, Norway), or CAE HPS (CAE, Sarasota, FL) are whole-task trainers that exhibit vital signs, variable airway features (eg, tongue swelling and laryngospasm), breathing patterns and sounds (eg, retractions to illustrate upper airway obstruction, breath sounds [wheezing], and pneumothorax), cardiovascular features (eg, heart sounds and peripheral pulses [diminished or absent]), and other relevant clinical findings (eg, abdominal sounds and distension, fontanelle bulging).[6] Incorporated into a simulated clinical setting outfitted with biomedical equipment and interprofessional health care teams, these mannequins can provide a high degree of clinical authenticity and realism to facilitate participants' engagement.

In addition to the development of simulators and task trainers for medical education, anesthesiology is widely credited with being the first health care specialty to target the avoidance of preventable harm. Based on research published on the causes of medical errors,[7] a substantial increase in malpractice costs in the 1980s led to a call for action. Under the leadership of Dr. Ellison C. Pierce, Jr., the President of the American Society of Anesthesiologists in 1984, the Anesthesia Patient Safety Foundation (APSF) was founded in 1985, which was committed to preventing harm from anesthesia.[8] In 1999, the Institute of Medicine (IOM) released "To Err Is Human: Building a Safer Health System," a widely cited report that estimated that 44,000 to 98,000 deaths occurred in the United States annually because of medical errors.[9] This report raised awareness of the impact of medical errors and emphasized patient safety challenges in the health care system, such as practitioners working independently in silo, stress owing to limited manpower, production pressure, lack of communication, and cognitive errors, all contributing to breakdowns and impinging on patient safety. The report pointed out that errors in human factors, the lack of teamwork, and the lack of a culture of safety were overarching components that resulted in adverse events in the health care industry.[9] Two main recommendations that the report made were: (1) "to make patient safety a priority corporate objective," and (2) "to create a learning environment."[9] The IOM report sent a powerful message that catalyzed national and international reforms in the health care industry to raise priorities in clinical care as well as education focused on patient safety.

Anesthesia crisis resource management (ACRM) was an outgrowth of the patient safety movement that began in anesthesia in the early 1980s when David Gaba and colleagues[10] at Stanford adapted the concepts from the aviation industry for medical education training. Concepts such as systematic training, rehearsal, performance assessment, and teamwork laid the foundations for ACRM, which was adapted from crew resource management in aviation terms.[10] Research grant funding from the APSF supported the early development of several forms of HPS. Further publicity and advocacy from APSF propelled anesthesiology to the forefront of specialties in the application and adoption of simulators, with strong patient safety implications through education, training, and research. Today, a substantial body of literature supports the value of teamwork for successful prevention of medical errors and the management of critical events.[11,12]

INTERPROFESSIONAL EDUCATION AND LEARNING

The subspecialty of otolaryngology anesthesia is distinctive in that the otolaryngologist and anesthesiologist literally work side by side and share overlapping patient anatomic and physiologic concerns.[13] The otolaryngology environment requires a unique collaboration between the anesthesiologist and surgeon to optimize patient care. Team training in the form of IPE and interprofessional learning (IPL) is critical for patient safety in the operating room in general, but more so in Ear/Nose/Throat (ENT) procedures requiring anesthesia, owing to the potential difficult airway and dynamic distortions of airway anatomy. Currently, simulation literature is focused on procedural skills in ENT or airway management, either for the surgeon or the anesthesia provider alone.[14,15] However, this individualized training is not sufficient for management of critical airway incidents in which crisis resource management and effective communication skills can affect patient safety. IPE refers to 2 or more professions learning with, from, and about each other to improve collaboration and the quality of care, whereas IPL is learning that arises from interaction between members of 2 or more professions (either as a result of IPE or spontaneously in the workplace).[16] One of the main goals of IPE is to create a highly trained, cohesive workforce that is ready to work with a team-oriented approach to provide patient-centered care.[17] In ENT anesthesia training, the incorporation of interprofessional learning between the anesthesiologist and otolaryngologist is particularly important because it promotes collaborative practice and interaction between the 2 professions. Promoting and fostering interprofessional learning that emphasizes constant and concise communication between the two professions is paramount to the safety of patients, and can be achieved by having the disciplines engaged in a high-fidelity simulation. To make the IPE exercise most effective, representatives from anesthesiology, otolaryngology, and nursing must all be present and participating, the objectives must be relevant to all parties and be made clear from the beginning, and the simulated scenario must engage all groups.[17] Immersive simulation can be achieved with a variety of simulators and technologies with varying levels of fidelity, including computerized high-fidelity physiologically modeled mannequins, standardized patients, and hybrid simulators. The next paragraphs discuss examples of airway skills that may require both anesthesiology and otolaryngology involvement, including management of aspirated foreign bodies, control of epistaxis, and difficult airway requiring a surgical airway using part-task trainers that have been modified and manipulated for the specific learning objective.

To create a foreign body in the airway model, a toy marble or food substance can be inserted into the oropharynx or trachea of a mannequin to create an exercise whereby both anesthesiology and ENT residents must practice managing the airway. Both specialties can practice manipulating the airway with appropriate instruments and communication of care during this simulated airway crisis.[18] Management of epistaxis can be another example whereby both providers must collaborate to manage the airway. By using a nasal cannula glued to the inside of a mannequin's nose, a simulation specialist can control the flow of "blood" through the tubing to simulate bleeding.[19,20] In the "can't ventilate, can't intubate" scenario, most anesthesiology and surgery residency programs train their learners separately using commercially available tracheotomy task trainers with cervical landmarks that can cause bleeding, resistance, and edema when cut into.[21] An interprofessional approach would be to combine this airway training session for both subspecialties to facilitate shared reflection and appreciation of the nuances of the difficult airway. Because an anesthesiology trainee would not normally be making a tracheostomy incision, having combined learning sessions with a surgical resident could provide an opportunity for discussion on how the actions of one provider can affect the other.

Using part-task airway and head-and-neck trainers in a collaborative training approach as described is a starting point to develop technical skills and can serve as an introduction to both IPE and IPL among the trainees of the 2 subspecialties. However, a real clinical situation involving an airway emergency or other head and neck disorder involves not only the anesthesiology and otolaryngology trainees, but also their respective attending physicians and nurses. Therefore, engineering a scenario using high-fidelity, whole-body, physiologically modeled mannequins with the multidisciplinary team can take the IPE and learning to another level. These interdisciplinary team simulations can occur in a simulation center, or in an in situ environment, such as a real patient room, emergency department, postanesthesia care unit, or operating room, as dictated by the scenario and learning objective. The in situ environment provides an extra level of fidelity, and provides the natural environment that the residents, attending physicians, and nurses find themselves in daily. Although in situ simulation seems ideal and can be used to investigate latent patient safety threats (eg, inadequate resources, environmental ergonomics), care must be taken to avoid introducing devices, fluids, and medication intended only for simulation use. For example, in New York, several patients inadvertently received "simulation-only" intravenous fluid and subsequently developed sepsis.[22] Although it was unclear how these items were introduced into the actual clinical environment, it is important to emphasize that "simulation-only" items must be labeled clearly and removed from real patient care settings. In addition, using actual operating rooms with representatives from ENT, anesthesiology, and nursing poses a logistical challenge and requires buy-in from perioperative leadership.

IN SITU INTERPROFESSIONAL TEAM TRAINING AND SYSTEMS IMPROVEMENT

This section discusses examples of programs that have incorporated multidisciplinary simulations into interprofessional team training and systems-based education. At Boston Children's Hospital, the department of otolaryngology introduced an in situ high-fidelity simulation program to teach teamwork, crisis resource management, and decision-making skills in airway management to a team of otolaryngology residents, anesthesia trainees, and operating room nurses.[23] At the Icahn School of Medicine at Mount Sinai, an in situ simulation was performed in preparation for an annual joint conference between the Anesthesiology and Otolaryngology departments. It took place in the operating room on the ENT floor and involved junior and senior anesthesiology residents, junior and senior otolaryngology residents, otolaryngology attending physicians, circulating nurses, and scrub technicians. For this case scenario, the CAE Apollo (CAE, Sarasota, FL), a high-fidelity wireless, whole-body simulator controlled remotely with a laptop computer was used. The clinical scenario involved a patient with a progressive obstructing airway mass and subsequent management of a difficult airway. Team dynamics was observed and recorded on video, and all participants underwent an internal debrief immediately following the simulation. An edited video was later shown at the joint conference to spark collaborative discussion and healthy, constructive criticism within and between both departments and operating room nursing staff.

In addition to enhancing resident education, IPE via multidisciplinary team simulations can help uncover latent errors in a medical system and improve patient safety. For instance, at Johns Hopkins, an interdisciplinary difficult airway response team was developed to manage hospital-wide airway emergencies. In situ simulation proved to be an invaluable tool to test systems, identify defects in resources and processes, and develop improvement strategies.[24]

ROLE OF SIMULATION IN THE FUTURE

Virtual reality and augmented reality have begun to enter health care, and its evolution is rapid. With virtual reality, the entire environment and everything within it is created: it does not exist in the real world. In contrast, with augmented reality, the environment is real and there are computer-generated images and sounds superimposed onto the real environment.

Virtual reality has already shown promising results in helping terminally ill patients with cancer with pain, tiredness, shortness of breath, and depression.[25] Virtual reality and augmented reality have long played a role in neurosurgery, where both modalities have helped neurosurgeons prepare for tumor excision and decision making for the best approach.[26] Some institutions have already implemented the use of virtual reality and augmented reality into medical student education. For example, these modalities are being used to teach anatomy and ultrasound imaging. Augmented reality adds layers of underlying muscles, tissues, blood vessels, and bone structures to the ultrasound images to better understand how to interpret these images. Some simulation centers have the ability to project hologram images of a patient over the HPS to make it more lifelike. The use of hologram images confers the ability to change the color of the HPS, such as blue lips resulting from hypoxia, which is otherwise one of the limitations of these high-fidelity whole-body simulators.[27]

As technology advances and cost decreases, virtual reality and augmented reality will become a bigger part of health care. The current virtual reality equipment and software allows for easy access, portability, and lower cost compared with a high-fidelity HPS. Many institutions cannot afford the cost of a high-fidelity simulator, yearly maintenance, and personnel to run the simulator. In addition to the cost of the simulator, to perform a multidisciplinary team simulation training exercise in an in situ environment, the time of each health care provider and utilization of the real clinical environment, along with use of real patient equipment, must be taken into account for the cost and feasibility of establishing such training environments. Virtual and augmented reality technology can substantially reduce or even eliminate some of these costs and will allow easier access to interdisciplinary simulation scenarios, such as an airway disaster or an airway fire scenario, between otolaryngologists, anesthesiologists, and nurses. The future of health care team training by virtual and augmented reality is to create multiplayer scenarios that individual providers can log into simultaneously under their respective roles (anesthesiologist, otolaryngologist, circulating nurse, scrub tech/nurse) from remote locations, at their convenience, and allow the high-fidelity scenario to unfold as they engage in IPE and learning. Furthermore, virtual and augmented reality technology will allow training of new health care providers as part of their onboarding process and also as part of their continuing and sustained education, regardless of the level of the provider (trainee, attending physician, junior or senior nurse).

SUMMARY

Even though the medical field was slow to accept simulation, a combination of increased emphasis on patient safety and focus on error prevention, as well as a shift toward an outcomes-based education model for medical education and training, has led simulation to be incorporated into every level of medical training. More importantly, at the graduate and postgraduate level, interdisciplinary and interprofessional education and learning via multidisciplinary team training is paramount in enhancing patient safety. Although all disciplines should partake in IPE/IPL, the intimate relationship between the otolaryngologist and anesthesiologist, and the high-stakes nature of the surgeries with potential loss of the airway, necessitates a collaborative simulation curriculum between these two subspecialties. For IPE and IPL to be most effective, representatives from nursing also need to be present for these simulation training sessions. In situ simulations can not only increase the level of fidelity of the scenario and enrich learners' engagement and participation, but also help diagnose latent errors and lead to the implementation of systematic process and workflow changes.

Technology is continuing to advance, and the future of virtual reality and augmented reality will make it possible for multidisciplinary simulation team training to take place at ever lowering costs.

REFERENCES

1. Frenk J, Chen L, Bhutta ZA, et al. Health professionals for a new century: transforming education to strengthen health systems in an interdependent world. Lancet 2010;376(9756):1923–58.
2. Rosen KR. The history of medical simulation. J Crit Care 2008;23(2):157–66.
3. Cooper JB, Taqueti VR. A brief history in the development of mannequin simulators for clinical education and training. Postgrad Med J 2008;84(997):563–70.
4. Bradley P. The history of simulation in medical education and possible future directions. Med Educ 2006;40(3):254–62.
5. Barrows HS, Abrahamson S. The programmed patient: a technique for appraising student performance in clinical neurology. J Med Educ 1964;39:802–5.
6. Schaefer JJ. Simulators and difficult airway management skills. Paediatr Anaesth 2004;14(1):28–37.
7. Cooper JB, Newbower RS, Long CD, et al. Preventable anesthesia mishaps: a study of human factors. Anesthesiology 1978;49:399–406.
8. The Anesthesia Patient Safety Foundation: "The establishment of the APSF" Pierce EC, Jr. Available at: http://www.apsf.org/about.php. Accessed March 2, 2019.
9. Kohn LT, Corrigan JM, Donaldson MS, editors. To err is human-building a safer health system. Washington, DC: National Academies Press; 2000. p. 312.
10. Gaba D, Howard S, Fish K, et al. Simulation-based training in anesthesia crisis resource management (ACRM): a decade of experience. Simul Gaming 2001; 32:175–93.
11. Gaba DM, DeAnda A. A comprehensive anesthesia simulation environment: recreating the operating room for research and training. Anesthesiology 1988; 69(3):387–94.
12. Gaba D, Fish K, Howard S. Crisis management in anesthesiology. Philadelphia: Churchill Livingstone; 1994.
13. Levine AI, DeMaria S, Govindaraj S. Working side by side: the important relationship between anesthesiologists and otolaryngologists. In: Levine AI, editor. Anesthesiology and otolaryngology. 1st edition. New York: Springer-Verlag; 2013. p. 1–2.
14. Musbahi O, Aydin A, Omran YA, et al. Current status of simulation in otolaryngology: a systematic review. J Surg Educ 2017;74(2):203–15.
15. Park CS. Simulation and quality improvement in anesthesiology. Anesthesiol Clin 2011;29(1):13–28.
16. Freeth D, Hammick M, Reeves S, et al. Effective interprofessional education: development, delivery and evaluation. Oxford (United Kingdom): Blackwell Publishing; 2005.
17. O'Brien RP, Mould J. Interprofessional education. In: Riley RH, editor. Manual of simulation in healthcare. Oxford (UK): Oxford University Press; 2016. p. 141–50.
18. Deutsch ES. High-fidelity patient simulation manikins to facilitate aerodigestive endoscopy training. Arch Otolaryngol Head Neck Surg 2008;134:625–9.
19. White ML, Ades A, Shefrin AE, et al. Task and procedural skills training. In: Grant VJ, Cheng A, editors. Comprehensive healthcare simulation: pediatrics. Springer International Publishing Switzerland; 2016. p. 139–52 [Chapter 11].

20. Deutsch ES, Javia LR. Simulation in otolaryngology. In: Levine AI, DeMaria S, Schwartz AD, Sim AJ, editors. The comprehensive textbook of healthcare simulation. New York: Springer-Verlag; 2014. p. 477–86 [Chapter 33].
21. John B, Suri I, Hillermann C, et al. Comparison of cricothyroidotomy on manikin vs. simulator: a randomized cross-over study. Anaesthesia 2007;62(10):1029–32.
22. New York Department of Health. Health advisory: improper use of simulation intravenous fluids not intended for human or animal use. Available at: https://apps.health.ny.gov/pub/ctrldocs/alrtview/postings/Notification_17915.pdf. Accessed March 29, 2003.
23. Volk MS, Ward J, Irias N, et al. Using medical simulation to teach crisis resource management and decision-making skills to otolaryngology housestaff. Otolaryngol Head Neck Surg 2011;145(1):35–42.
24. Mark LJ, Herzer KR, Cover R, et al. Difficult airway response team: a novel quality improvement program for managing hospital-wide airway emergencies. Anesth Analg 2015;121:127–39.
25. Niki K, Okamoto Y, Maeda I, et al. A novel palliative care approach using virtual reality for improving various symptoms of terminal cancer patients: a preliminary prospective, multicenter study. J Palliat Med 2019;22(6):702–7.
26. Lee C, Wong GKC. Virtual reality and augmented reality in the management of intracranial tumors: a review. J Clin Neurosci 2019;62:14–20.
27. Breining G. Future or fad? Virtual reality in medical education. AAMCNews 2018. Available at: news.aamc.org/medical-education/article/future-or-fad-virtual-reality-medical-education/.

Patient Safety in Anesthesia

Ellen S. Deutsch, MD, MS, CPPS, FSSH[a],*, Tracey Straker, MD, MS, MPH, CBA[b]

KEYWORDS

- Foreign body aspiration • Airway fire • Laryngospasm • Difficult airway
- Hemorrhage • Safety-II • Simulation • Resilience engineering

KEY POINTS

- Anesthesiologists and otolaryngologists share the airway.
- Potential complications of otolaryngologic surgery include airway fires, hemorrhage, airway obstruction, wrong-site procedures, and local anesthetic toxicity.
- Contemporary approaches to optimize patient safety include resilience engineering, application of Safety-II principles, and simulation.

INTRODUCTION

This article reviews key patient safety topics of concern to both anesthesiologists and otolaryngologists including initiatives to prevent operating room fires, difficult airway misadventures, and wrong-site surgery. Topics are presented alongside initiatives to mitigate risk. Also discussed are key concepts of patient safety and how they can apply to otolaryngology patients.

ONCE UPON A TIME...A TRUE STORY

A young child arrived in the Emergency Department (ED) with a history of tripping while eating sunflower seeds. The incident was immediately followed by a coughing fit and then persistent noisy breathing. In the ED, continuous pulse oximetry demonstrated oxygen saturation in the high 80s (abnormally low). The history combined with the physical examination findings was suggestive of foreign body aspiration.

The patient was brought to the operating room for endoscopic removal of the suspected foreign body. This procedure is usually performed by instrumenting the airway during intermittent periods of apnea interspersed with episodes of ventilation. In preparation for the procedure, the anesthesiologist provided mask ventilation with

Disclosure Statement: No disclosures.
[a] Anesthesiology and Critical Care, Department of Anesthesiology and Critical Care Medicine, University of Pennsylvania Perelman School of Medicine, Children's Hospital of Philadelphia, Room 9NW9329, 3401 Civic Center Boulevard, Philadelphia, PA 19104, USA; [b] Department of Anesthesiology, Montefiore Medical Center, The University Hospital for Albert Einstein College of Medicine, 110 East 210th Street, 4th Floor Silver Zone, Bronx, NY 10467, USA
* Corresponding author.
E-mail address: deutsches@email.chop.edu

supplemental oxygen. Preoxygenation to an oxygen saturation of 100% would provide an oxygen reserve to optimize and prolong the opportunity for endoscopy. In this case, the patient's oxygen saturation remained lower than 90% despite active attempts to ventilate and oxygenate the patient.

The otolaryngologist and the anesthesiologist conferred about the risks of proceeding with endoscopy despite unfavorable oxygen saturation levels, versus the risks of not proceeding with endoscopy. If endoscopy did not proceed, the patient's airway obstruction would not be alleviated. After discussing how to optimize their interaction to minimize the duration of apneic periods, they proceeded with endoscopy using a ventilating bronchoscope containing a telescope, which allowed the anesthesiologist to attempt ventilation via the bronchoscope.

Once the bronchoscope was passed into the trachea, pink frothy liquid was seen. The anesthesiologist provided positive pressure ventilation, which temporarily dispersed the fluid, allowing visualization of sunflower seed fragments obstructing both main bronchi. An optical forceps, which provides illuminated visualization, was used to remove the foreign body fragments. However, this equipment interfered with the ability to ventilate the patient, so the otolaryngologist and the anesthesiologist rapidly alternated their management of the airway, including alternating their spatial relationship at the head of the patient. Using this coordinated process, the fragments were successfully removed, adequate ventilation was accomplished, and the patient's oxygen saturation levels returned to normal.

The care for this patient was successful because the anesthesiologist and the otolaryngologist "shared the airway" in a deliberate "ballet." They developed a shared mental model, and each appreciated the role, skills, and requirements of the other. Their communication facilitated coordinated efforts to achieve the most effective and safest care for the patient.

PATIENT SAFETY HAZARDS COMMON TO ANESTHESIOLOGISTS AND OTOLARYNGOLOGISTS
Collaboration to Prevent Airway Fires

There are other patient safety hazards that otolaryngologists and anesthesiologists uniquely face together as they share the airway, such as airway fires. Data from Pennsylvania demonstrate that the majority of reported surgical fires affect the scalp, face, or neck of patients.[1] Otolaryngology surgeries are among the procedures that provide the greatest risk of airway fire because of the close proximity of all 3 components of the fire triad.[2] In procedures such as tonsillectomies, electrocautery (an ignition source) may be used millimeters away from an endotracheal tube (fuel) in an oxygen-enriched environment. Managing the well-known triad of fuel, oxidizer, and ignition source is the collective responsibility of the operating room team.

A team-based time-out before surgery can mitigate the risk of airway fire. During the time-out, the surgical plan, potential ignition sources, oxygen requirements of the patient, and available safety resources such as water on the surgical field should be discussed.[2]

During the procedure, the fraction of inspired oxygen (Fio_2) should be less than 30%, if the patient's pulmonary function can tolerate that level of support. The risk of airway fire increases if the Fio_2 is greater than 30%.[2] The risk also increases if oxygen is delivered in an open fashion, such as by nasal cannula, as opposed to delivery via a closed system such as a cuffed endotracheal tube (ETT). ETT closed oxygen delivery is considered more secure than delivery of oxygen by open systems, or even by a supraglottic device, because the cuff is inflated below the cords, thereby creating a barrier and closed space for the oxygen delivery. Nitrous oxide is also a flammable gas,[3] and, as with oxygen, its use should be minimized in otolaryngology procedures that use an ignition source. For oropharyngeal procedures, the use of metal-tip suction in the oropharynx to remove gases that may leak around the ETT is encouraged.[2]

Endoscopic surgery with an ETT and laser accompanied by an oxygen concentration higher than 30% provides the components of another classic clinical "fire triad." The ETT can become the fuel ignited by the laser in an oxygen-rich environment. Cowles[4] recommends that endoscopic laser surgery be performed with a cuffed laser-safe ETT, or without an ETT (eg, during apneic periods), and that the laser fiber tip be placed more than 1 cm from the tip of the bronchoscope. If an airway fire occurs, burning material should be quickly removed from the airway, the oxygen source disconnected from the patient, and the surgical field flooded with water. These 3 steps occur within seconds of each other.[4]

Tracheostomy surgery carries its own inherent risk of airway fire, because these patients often have increased oxygen requirements. Hemostasis should be achieved before entering the airway. Ignition sources such as electrocautery should be avoided, and instruments such as scalpels with no heat element (cold instruments) should be used to incise the trachea.[2]

Anesthetics for facial plastic surgery may use open oxygen-delivery techniques, such as nasal cannulas or face masks, which can result in pooling of oxygen near the surgical field. Depending on the pulmonary function of the patient, the type of surgery, and the type of sedation used, it may be possible to deliver safe and effective sedation without the addition of supplemental oxygen. If the patient does not tolerate a "room air anesthetic" and supplemental oxygen is needed, conversion to a closed oxygen-delivery system via ETT or supraglottic device should be considered.[5]

Sharing Airway Management

The nature of the surgical procedure determines the anesthetic approach. Specific otolaryngology procedures may benefit from an inhalational induction with patients breathing spontaneously, despite the risk of laryngospasm. Laryngospasm is defined as the sustained closure of the vocal folds resulting in obstructive apnea.[6] Oral and pharyngeal spaces shared by anesthesiologists and otolaryngologists, such as for tonsillectomy and adenoidectomy, incur the highest risk of laryngospasm.[7] Recognition of patients at higher risk of laryngospasm enables the anesthesiologist to acquire an adequate depth of anesthesia during both induction and emergence.[2]

Anesthetic management for tracheobronchial surgeries, such as laryngotracheal reconstruction (LTR), is particularly challenging. The anesthesiology provider and surgeon take turns managing the airway, sometimes in rapid sequence and with limited physical control. Communication between the anesthesiologist and the otolaryngologist is essential. Areas of the LTR that require a "ballet" between the anesthesiologist and the otolaryngologist include ventilation of the distal portion of the trachea while the proximal trachea is open, and during emergence from anesthesia. If a guardian suture has been placed, securing the submental crease to the anterior chest wall to prevent excessive hyperextension of the neck, it must be protected.[8]

Anesthesiologists and otolaryngologists collaborate as members of difficult airway response teams (DARTs), multidisciplinary teams that also include critical care providers. DARTs are tasked with securing failing or lost airways outside the operating room. A failed airway or lost airway occurs when there is an inability to intubate the patient and an inability to oxygenate the patient adequately using bag mask ventilation or a supraglottic device.[9] In emergent circumstances, front-of-neck access via cricothyrotomy is the recommended procedure for the anesthesiologist.[10] Otolaryngologists may resort to cricothyrotomy or tracheostomy. The "maiden" DART, established in 2013 at Johns Hopkins University, has performed more than 1000 airway interventions, with no adverse airway outcomes.[11]

Coordination to Prevent Wrong-Site Procedures

Wrong-site surgery is defined as surgery performed on the wrong body part, wrong side of the body, wrong patient, or at the wrong level of the correctly identified anatomic site. This definition includes nonsurgical invasive procedures such as regional anesthetic blocks, and dermatologic, obstetric, and dental procedures.[12] According to The Joint Commission, wrong-site surgery is the third most common sentinel event after falls and unintended retention of a foreign body[13]; wrong-site procedures occur about once a week in Pennsylvania.[14] In a study by Stahel and colleagues,[15] common causes for wrong-site procedures were errors in judgment (85.0%) and the lack of calling for a time-out (72.0%).

In 2008, the World Health Organization (WHO) instituted the Global Patient Safety Challenge, "Safe Surgery Saves Lives." The program includes a checklist, which has 3 components (**Fig. 1**):[16]

- Sign in (before induction of anesthesia)
- Time-out (after induction and before surgical incision)
- Sign out (during or immediately after wound closure but before removing the patient from the operating room)

The WHO reports that their checklist has decreased morbidity and mortality.[16]

In all documentation involving a bilateral organ, the laterality of the organ should be named. Anatomic marking of the surgical site is only performed by the attending surgeon, and verbal confirmation of the site and procedure with the patient should take place before the patient is brought into the operating room.[17]

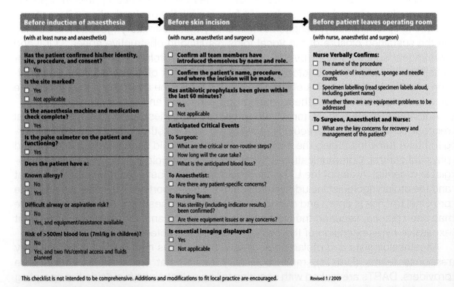

Fig. 1. World Health Organization surgical safety checklist. (*From* World Health Organization (WHO). WHO Surgical Safety Checklist, 2009. Available at: https://www.who.int/patientsafety/safesurgery/checklist/en/; with permission.)

Cooperation to Manage Hemorrhage

Severe bleeding or massive hemorrhage is a rare but possibly deadly event that may be seen in the perioperative arena, operating room, intensive care unit, and postanesthesia care unit.

A 2014 analysis of data from the Anesthesia Closed Claims Database suggested that inadequate communication and lack of organized protocols were key missing components that might have mitigated adverse outcomes related to hemorrhage.[18] Lack of timely diagnosis of blood loss, lack of timely transfusion, and lack of timely return to the operating room were common factors. Among claims including lack of communication, 60% involved hemorrhage.[18]

Usually otolaryngology procedures have minimal blood loss, but head and neck procedures, such as thyroidectomy, neck dissection, and major head and neck cancer resections, particularly radical maxillectomy, have the potential for significant blood loss because large vascular structures are often in or near the surgical field. Team communication, training of operating room personnel using simulation, and clinical drills have been shown to improve team performance. The Massive Transfusion Protocol, a prearranged grouping of blood products activated by one phone call, demonstrates team communication and organization via protocol.[19]

Tonsillectomy is one of the most common otolaryngology surgeries performed, with 700,000 operations taking place in the United States annually.[20] Post-tonsillectomy hemorrhage (PTH) is a feared complication that can require readmission and return to the operating room,[21] and can be fatal. The incidence of primary PTH, which occurs within the first 24 hours after surgery, is 0.2% to 2.2%, and the incidence of secondary PTH is 0.1% to 4.8%. Most incidents of secondary hemorrhage occur within 2 weeks following surgery.[20,22] PTH is an emergent situation that must be dealt with in a timely manner. Challenges that might be encountered by the anesthesiologist include a presumptive full stomach (which may increase the risk of aspiration), severe dehydration, and tachycardia. Management usually includes fluid resuscitation, rapid sequence induction, and laryngoscopy with insertion of a cuffed ETT.[23]

Preparations to Manage "Difficult Airways"

Physical or physiologic conditions (eg, neck trauma) can create conditions that make controlling an individual patient's airway particularly challenging. Awake intubation can be used to manage a patient with an anticipated difficult airway. Multiple techniques and pharmacologic "concoctions" may be used to deliver a dense and functional local anesthetic (LA) block. LA, particularly using lidocaine, can be applied topically or injected to provide local or regional anesthesia to facilitate awake intubation. Topical laryngeal and tracheal LA can be administered by nebulizer, although this may result in a "patchy" block. Injected regional airway blocks allow the clinician to be certain of the amount of LA given.

Each LA has a defined dosage per kilogram recommended to prevent local anesthetic systemic toxicity (LAST). LAST is a systemic complication of LA that includes both cardiovascular and neurologic toxicity, which may be evidenced by seizures.[24] Management includes administration of intralipids.[24]

Excessive amounts of LA, particularly benzocaine, lidocaine, and prilocaine, can also cause methemoglobinemia.[25] Methemoglobin is a form of hemoglobin in which the ferrous (Fe^{2+}) irons of heme are oxidized to the ferric (Fe^{3+}) state. The ferric hemes of methemoglobin are unable to reversibly bind oxygen, so oxygenation of end organs is compromised.[25] Cyanosis in the presence of normal partial arterial pressure of oxygen (Pao_2) should raise the suspicion of methemoglobinemia. Diagnosis may be confirmed by co-oximetry of an arterial blood gas. Methylene blue and ascorbic acid are used to treat methemoglobinemia and should be readily available.[25]

Addressing Comorbidities

In recent years, comorbidities such as obstructive sleep apnea (OSA) and obesity have spawned numerous protocols intended to improve the safety of perioperative management of affected patients. OSA is a chronic syndrome characterized by periodic partial or complete obstruction in the upper airway during sleep.[26] Airway surgery in the presence of OSA may increase perioperative risk, depending in part on the invasiveness and nature of the surgery, and the type of anesthetic.[27]

Risk-reduction strategies include preoperative assessment using the STOP-BANG instrument, intraoperative management with multimodal pain reduction options when applicable, and postoperative physiologic monitoring. The STOP-BANG questionnaire, an 8-question validated tool, has become one of the most common instruments for preoperative assessment of patients with documented and undocumented OSA.[28] Intraoperative management with judicious use of opioids and postoperative monitoring with continuous pulse oximetry are recommended for patients with OSA by the American Society of Anesthesiologists.[27]

Assessing Upper Airway Patency

Inadequate knowledge of the anatomy of the patient scheduled for tracheostomy, laryngectomy, or laryngotracheal separation may result in significant morbidity and mortality. Understanding the difference between a tracheostomy and a laryngectomy or laryngotracheal separation stoma is critical. Because a laryngectomy involves removing the larynx, the laryngectomy stoma is not connected to the upper airway; a patient who has undergone a laryngectomy cannot be intubated orally in an airway emergency. In laryngotracheal separation procedures, the trachea is disconnected from the upper airway; although the larynx is not removed, there is a similar inability to intubate orally. By contrast, it may be possible to intubate a tracheostomy patient orally, although it may be difficult. Communication between all services taking care of patients after tracheostomy, laryngectomy, or laryngotracheal separation is crucial. One approach to the management of tracheostomy and stoma patients was developed by European organizations in 2012.[29] They advocated for communication to all services taking care of patients with tracheal stomas, including color-coordinated signs with detailed information regarding type of surgery and patency of the upper airway, placed above the patient's bed so that anyone managing a patient's airway could clearly understand the anatomy.[29] Information that accompanies the patient, such as a wrist band with medical information, might also be helpful.

TRADITIONAL SAFETY PROCESSES
Making Health Care Safer

Over the past 2 decades, attention to patient safety has gained momentum. Patient and family expectations for safe care have increased, and our understanding of processes that support safety has improved. Safety is an emergent property, which means that it arises from a combination of factors. One way to conceptualize the contributory factors is with the SEIPS 2.0 model of sociotechnical systems.[30] This model describes a work system that has individuals (both patients and providers) at the center, interacting with tasks, tools, and technologies, the organization, and internal and external environments. The work system interacts with work processes, which may be physical, cognitive, social, or behavioral; the work system also interacts with work outcomes. For example, the outcome of a surgical or anesthetic intervention may influence how a similar patient-care challenge is approached in the future. The components of sociotechnical systems have dynamic relationships, and feedback loops contribute to intended and unintended adaptations.[30]

In the foreign body aspiration event described earlier, the anesthesiologist and otolaryngologist developed a coordinated plan during an urgent situation. This relationship is based on a mutual expertise, their experience working with each other, and deliberate discussions. Providers with less general experience, and less experience working with each other, would benefit from purposeful discussions of hazards, and potential mitigation strategies, before providing patient care together. A formal implementation of this process could be constructed as a failure mode effects analysis (FMEA).[31] Because there are infinite ways that a patient may be harmed, FMEAs are intended to help prioritize harm-prevention efforts. **Fig. 2** shows a grid that combines information about the potential impact and the anticipated frequency of an event or condition that may cause harm. Items that have higher scores are prioritized for mitigation. Although FMEAs are usually applied to system hazards, the principles are relevant for individual cases. The application of FMEAs for individual cases is often less formal.

FMEA is generally used in a proactive manner, whereas root cause analysis (RCA) is generally implemented in response to an adverse patient-care event. As the name implies, the objective is to understand the root, or roots, of the adverse event. The RCA process was an advance in understanding adverse events, because it acknowledges the importance of factors preceding the final act of commission or omission associated with an adverse outcome. Apparent cause analysis (a less intensive investigation) and common cause analysis (aggregating results of multiple RCAs)[2,32] are variations of RCAs. It is difficult to avoid hindsight bias about the decisions or actions taken to care for a patient when conducting an RCA because the outcome of the interventions are known.[33]

The Importance of Reporting

Another way to collect information for safety enhancement is by implementing an event-reporting system. Reporting systems usually incorporate demographic information about the patient, a taxonomy of types of patient-care events, and a taxonomy of harm or outcome. There is usually an opportunity for a free-text description of some aspects of the patient-care event. A variety of patient-care event-type taxonomies have been published[34–37]; many organizations use an event-type taxonomy based on the Agency for Healthcare Research and Quality common formats.[38]

Patient harm may range from a minor temporary injury to a serious injury with temporary or permanent harm, or death. It is useful to collect information about "near-miss" events, in which harm was prevented from reaching a patient, as well as "unsafe

		Frequency			
		Rare	Uncommon	Common	Frequent
Severity	Minimal	1	2	3	4
	Moderate	2	4	6	8
	Severe	3	6	9	12
	Catastrophic	4	8	12	16

Fig. 2. Example of a failure mode effects analysis (FMEA) calculation grid, which allows prioritization scores to be assigned based on the frequency and severity of patient safety hazards. Some FMEAs also include detectability as a consideration.

conditions," in which a patient-care hazard is an identified event before it is related to a specific patient (eg, a medication shortage). Reporting near misses and unsafe conditions provides opportunities to mitigate hazards before patients are harmed, and may provide information about interventions that were effective in preventing patient harm.

The criteria for reporting events determine the sort of information that may be collected. Reporting based only on error requires a preliminary assumption that someone has made a mistake; it is noteworthy that patients sometimes sustain harm even if no one has made a mistake during their care. If reporting based on error includes a condition of deviating from accepted standards, the reporting will focus on the "sharp end" or "coalface" providers. However, if the objective of reporting is to improve safety, reporting based on harm (or potential harm), rather than error, provides a broader perspective on patient safety events.

Simulation and Patient Safety

Various types of simulation can be helpful in understanding how harm occurred or was prevented. Often simulation is considered a method to teach or test individuals or teams, but it also has applications in understanding and improving patient-care systems. Re-enacting patient-care events in situ (in actual patient-care locations, using actual patient-care equipment) can reveal conditions that may not have surfaced during individual or group interviews, such as during an RCA. For example, re-enacting a medication-dose error that occurred during the use of an infusion pump revealed that the numeric keys on the pump registered digits twice (eg, 2 became 22) for multiple users, suggesting a technical problem with the equipment. Simulation involving individuals or teams can also be used to explore potential solutions when hazards have been identified. Incorporating care providers who will be involved in implementing potential solutions has multiple benefits, including the opportunity to test solutions without direct risk to patients, incorporate the wisdom and experience of the providers, and engage providers so that they have ownership of the solution.

It is not necessary to wait for an adverse patient-care event before implementing simulation to assess patient-care systems. System hazards may be serendipitously identified during simulations, particularly simulations conducted in situ, even if the simulations were intended for other purposes, such as education or research. System hazards may also be the planned focus of the simulation or may be intentionally sought during the debriefing occurring after the simulation. System hazards identified during simulations have the same importance as hazards identified by other means, and should be reported through the organization's hazard reporting system to receive appropriate organizational prioritization and attention.

How Can Resilience Engineering Principles Help?

The resources and processes required to provide safe patient care are constantly evolving, both at the level of the individual patient's needs and at larger system levels (and at all the levels in between). Providing safe care under these dynamic conditions requires resilience. Resilience is defined by Wears and colleagues as "...the ability of the health care system to adjust its functioning prior to, during, or following events (changes, disturbances, opportunities) and thereby sustain required operations under both expected and unexpected conditions."[39]

Resilience engineering principles provide a framework to better understand health care, and support conditions that may allow safe health care to emerge. First, health care delivery is a complex adaptive system, which means that no individual can ever know the system completely. Complexity is a feature of the system as a whole, not necessarily of the components inside the system. Processes and relationships are fluid and dynamic, and environmental conditions are constantly evolving.[40–44]

Within health care delivery, health care providers (agents) constantly act, and constantly react to the actions of other agents. Health care providers must continually adjust how they work, because work conditions are underspecified, or incompletely understandable, and because interventions may have unpredictable consequences. These concepts apply at multiple system levels, including the level of macro systems at or beyond the organizational level, and at the level of departmental or patient-care units. They also apply at the level of caring for individual patients with limitless combinations of medical conditions and preferences.[40–44] Health care delivery is a human-made system integrated into a natural system as a subsystem.[45] Despite prodigious knowledge of human anatomy, physiology, and pathology, many mysteries remain.

Safe management of patients requires many skills, including the capacity to adapt to unknown or evolving patient characteristics. This ability to adapt is a component or perhaps a consequence of resilience. At the system level, Hollnagel and colleagues[46] have characterized resilience as including the following capacities:

- Monitor: know what to look for; includes being sensitive to "weak signals" or off-nominal events
- Respond: know what to do; includes having the ability to adapt responses to diverse circumstances
- Learn: know what has happened; includes understanding events that have occurred or are occurring
- Anticipate: know what to expect; includes understanding the progression and consequences of actions or conditions

Woods[47] describes the absence of resilience as brittleness, which includes an inability to absorb or adapt, or a lack of buffering capacity. If care is given close to a performance boundary (eg, at the threshold of harm), lack of resilience may be demonstrated by a lack of margin to accommodate physiologic stresses. Intolerant systems, including physiologic systems, will collapse when pressure exceeds adaptive capacity, rather than degrading gracefully.[47]

These characteristics of resilience systems are often described at the system level, but they have applicability to the care of patient populations and individual patients, and the capacity for resilient behavior may be a component of effective collaboration between anesthesiologists and otolaryngologists.

Similarly, threats to patient well-being can be considered using resilience engineering constructs. "Regular" threats occur frequently enough that providers develop standard responses. An intraoperative example might be oxygen desaturation, or a cardiac arrhythmia. "Irregular" threats are unexpected but not impossible or unimaginable; they require self-organization and improvisation. An intraoperative example might be laceration of a major vessel or an equipment malfunction. The third type of threat is an "unexampled event," which is so awful or unexpected that it requires more than the improvisation necessary for an irregular threat. Almost by definition an unexampled threat cannot be prospectively identified, but such a threat might equate to a tornado or aircraft hitting a hospital.

Safety-I and Safety-II: Complementary Approaches

So how can we keep patients safe amid innumerable threats? The more traditional approach to patient safety, sometimes called "Safety-I," has been to define safety by its opposite: failure. Failure is thought to be preventable by having people behave as expected and trained, and accidents arise from variability. Safety comes from limiting and constraining providers via standardization, procedures, rules, and barriers. Investigations of failures have a critical tone. Even if the investigators are enlightened enough to understand that the failure is not solely the responsibility of the individual at the sharp end, there is often a search for an error made by an individual proximal to the sharp end.[48]

Safety-II complements (but does not replace) Safety-I. In Safety-II principles, safe patient care is defined by its goal: success. Providers have to be able to adjust behavior and interpret procedures. Harm is a result of incomplete adaptation, and safety arises from supporting the provider by making boundaries, hazards, and goal conflicts visible. Safety is enhanced by developing a repertoire of potential responses. There is value is seeking to understand why most patient care goes well, and the tone of inquiry is appreciative.

Safety-I and Safety-II are complementary, and both perspectives have appropriate applications. Vincent and Amalberti[49] have defined a range of potential processes that align well with Safety-I and Safety-II principles. They describe three contrasting approaches to safety, ranging from strict standardization to expert-derived adaptation, based on the nature of the patient-care context. The following concepts are adapted from the principles addressing contrasting approaches to safety as stated by Vincent and Amalberti[49]:

1. Avoid risk: Examples include blood transfusion; risk is excluded with regulations and supervision; power is held by regulators and supervisors; prevention strategies are prioritized
2. Manage risk: Examples include scheduled surgery; risk is not sought but is inherent in the processes; power is held by the group; risk is minimized by protocols and adaptation strategies
3. Embrace risk: Examples include mass casualties and infrastructure failures; risk is inherent and unavoidable; power is held by experts; risk is managed by adaptation and recovery

Humans Are Assets

Finally, humans are essential components of safe and effective health care delivery. In addition to understanding human physiology, health care providers must also manage increasingly complex relationships with automation and escalating societal expectations.[50] Humans have situational awareness—the capacity to perceive, comprehend, and project[51]—that is necessary to guide technologic and other advances. Humans have the ability to make sense in complex environments, which allows us to make decisions and set goals.

As anesthesiologists and otolaryngologists we may have the closest relationship of any physician dyads, but we also rely on, and should appreciate, the expertise and dedication of nurses, technicians, and an often underappreciated but large variety of supporting professionals with other skills who also contribute to safe health care. The Institute of Medicine (now the National Academy of Medicine) describes people working in health care as "among the most educated and dedicated work force in any industry."[52] Anesthesiologists and otolaryngologists are essential assets and sources of creativity and solutions: we learn and improve ourselves, our teams, and the complex systems we work within; we invent, create, and develop health care advances and solutions; we offer empathy and compassion; and we provide ever-improving health care.[53]

SUMMARY

Patient safety in head and neck surgery depends on communication and a team-based approach. Otolaryngologists and anesthesiologists, as well as nurses, other health care professionals, and support staff, must work together as a seamless unit to ensure patient safety. Appreciating, educating, and supporting anesthesiologists and otolaryngologists, and the teams they work with, will allow provision of the safest possible health care. Continuing medical education, team-based approaches dedicated to patient safety, communication between providers, reporting adverse events and hazards, and implementing quality improvement initiatives will support an ongoing elegant, safe "airway ballet."

REFERENCES

1. Bruley ME, Arnold TV, Finley E, et al. Surgical fires: decreasing incidence relies on continued prevention efforts. Pa Patient Saf Advis 2018;15(2). Available at: http://patientsafety.pa.gov/ADVISORIES/Pages/201806_SurgicalFires.aspx.

2. Smith LP, Roy S, editors. OR fire safety video commentary for the ENT surgeon. Rochester (MN): Anesthesia Patient Safety Foundation; 2019. Available at: https://www.apsf.org/videos/or-fire-safety-video/or-fire-safety-video-commentary-for-the-ent-surgeon/.

3. Orhan-Sungur M, Komatsu R, Sherman A, et al. Effect of nasal cannula oxygen administration on oxygen concentration at facial and adjacent landmarks. Anaesthesia 2009;64(5):521-6.

4. Cowles CEJ, editor. Fire safety in the operating room. Philadelphia (PA): UpToDate Wolters Kluwer; 2019.

5. Feldman JM, Stoelting RK, editors. OR fire safety video commentary for the anesthesia professional. Rochester (MN): Anesthesia Patient Safety Foundation; 2019.

6. Gavel G, Walker RWM. Laryngospasm in anaesthesia. Continuing Education in Anaesthesia Critical Care & Pain 2013;14(2):47-51.

7. Vlok R, Melhuish TM, Chong C, et al. Adjuncts to local anaesthetics in tonsillectomy: a systematic review and meta-analysis. J Anesth 2017;31(4):608-16.

8. Ahuja S, Cohen B, Hinkelbein J, et al. Practical anesthetic considerations in patients undergoing tracheobronchial surgeries: a clinical review of current literature. J Thorac Dis 2016;8(11):3431-41.

9. Brown CAI, Walls RM. The emergency airway algorithms. In: Brown CAI, Sakles JC, Mick NW, editors. The Walls manual of emergency airway management. 5th edition. Philadelphia (PA): Wolters Kluwer; 2017. p. 25.

10. Apfelbaum JL, Hagberg CA, Caplan RA, et al. Practice guidelines for management of the difficult airway: an updated report by the American Society of Anesthesiologists task force on management of the difficult airway. Anesthesiology 2013;118(2):251-70.

11. Mark L, Lester L, Cover R, et al. A decade of difficult airway response team: lessons learned from a hospital-wide difficult airway response team program. Crit Care Clin 2018;34(2):239-51.

12. Hanchanale V, Rao AR, Motiwala H, et al. Wrong site surgery! how can we stop it? Urol Ann 2014;6(1):57-62.

13. Summary data of sentinel events reviewed by the joint commission. 2019. Available at: https://www.jointcommission.org/assets/1/6/Summary_4Q_2018.pdf. Accessed May 27, 2019.

14. Patient safety topics: wrong-site surgery. 2019. Available at: http://patientsafety.pa. gov/pst/Pages/Wrong%20Site%20Surgery/hm.aspx?psapst=Wrong-Site Surgery#. Accessed May 27, 2019.

15. Stahel PF, Sabel AL, Victoroff MS, et al. Wrong-site and wrong-patient procedures in the universal protocol era: analysis of a prospective database of physician self-reported occurrences. Arch Surg 2010;145(10):978–84.

16. Patient safety WHO surgical safety checklist. 2019. Available at: https://www.who. int/patientsafety/safesurgery/checklist/en/.

17. Knight N, Aucar J. Use of an anatomic marking form as an alternative to the universal protocol for preventing wrong site, wrong procedure and wrong person surgery. Am J Surg 2010;200(6):803–7.

18. Dutton RP, Lee LA, Stephens LS, et al. Massive hemorrhage: a report from the anesthesia closed claims project. Anesthesiology 2014;121(3):450–8.

19. Kutcher ME, Kornblith LZ, Narayan R, et al. A paradigm shift in trauma resuscitation: evaluation of evolving massive transfusion practices. JAMA Surg 2013; 148(9):834–40.

20. Goldman JL, Baugh RF, Davies L, et al. Mortality and major morbidity after tonsillectomy: Etiologic factors and strategies for prevention. Laryngoscope 2013; 123(10):2544–53. Available at: http://elinks.library.upenn.edu/?sid=OVID: medline&id=pmid:23595509.

21. Odhagen E, Sunnergren O, Soderman AH, et al. Reducing post-tonsillectomy haemorrhage rates through a quality improvement project using a Swedish national quality register: a case study. Eur Arch Otorhinolaryngol 2018;275(6): 1631–9.

22. Wall JJ, Tay K. Postoperative tonsillectomy hemorrhage. Emerg Med Clin North Am 2018;36(2):415–26.

23. Bangera A. Anaesthesia for adenotonsillectomy: an update. Indian J Anaesth 2017;61(2):103–9.

24. Regional and topical anesthesia for awake endotracheal intubation. 2019. Available at: https://www.nysora.com/techniques/head-and-neck-blocks/airway/ regional-topical-anesthesia-awake-endotracheal-intubation/.

25. Prchal JT, editor. Clinical features, diagnosis, and treatment of methemoglobinemia. Philadelphia (PA): Wolters Kluwer; 2018.

26. Spence DL, Han T, McGuire J, et al. Obstructive sleep apnea and the adult perioperative patient. J Perianesth Nurs 2015;30(6):528–45.

27. American Society of Anesthesiologists Task Force on Perioperative Management of patients with obstructive sleep apnea. Practice guidelines for the perioperative management of patients with obstructive sleep apnea: an updated report by the American Society of Anesthesiologists task force on perioperative management of patients with obstructive sleep apnea. Anesthesiology 2014;120(2):268–86.

28. Chung F, Abdullah HR, Liao P. STOP-bang questionnaire: a practical approach to screen for obstructive sleep apnea. Chest 2016;149(3):631–8.

29. McGrath BA, Bates L, Atkinson D, et al. Multidisciplinary guidelines for the management of tracheostomy and laryngectomy airway emergencies. Anaesthesia 2012;67(9):1025–41.

30. Holden RJ, Carayon P, Gurses AP, et al. SEIPS 2.0: a human factors framework for studying and improving the work of healthcare professionals and patients. Ergonomics 2013;56(11):1669–86.

31. The basics of healthcare failure mode and effect analysis. 2019. Available at: https://www.patientsafety.va.gov/professionals/onthejob/hfmea.asp.

32. National Patient Safety Foundation. RCA2: improving root cause analyses and actions to prevent harm. Boston (MA): National Patient Safety Foundation and Institute for Healthcare Improvement; 2015.

33. Dekker S, Hollnagel E, Woods DD, et al. Resilience engineering: new directions for measuring and maintaining safety in complex systems. Final report, 2008. Lund University School of Aviation.

34. World Health Organization. Patient safety the conceptual framework for the international classification for patient safety. World Health Organization; 2019.

35. Chang A, Schyve PM, Croteau RJ, et al. The JCAHO patient safety event taxonomy: a standardized terminology and classification schema for near misses and adverse events. Int J Qual Health Care 2005;17(2):95–105.

36. De Ville K, Novick LF. Toward a taxonomy of public health error. J Public Health Manag Pract 2010;16(3):216–20.

37. Hillin E, Hicks RW. Medication errors from an emergency room setting: safety solutions for nurses. Crit Care Nurs Clin North Am 2010;22(2):191–6.

38. Patient safety organization (PSO) program common formats. Available at: https://www.pso.ahrq.gov/common.

39. Wears RL, Hollnagel E, Braithwaite J. Resilient health care vol. 2: the resilience of everyday clinical work. Abingdon (Oxon): Ashgate; 2015.

40. Clay-Williams R, Hounsgaard J, Hollnagel E. Where the rubber meets the road: Using FRAM to align work-as-imagined with work-as-done when implementing clinical guidelines. Implement Sci 2015;10:125.

41. Dekker S. Drift into failure from hunting broken components to understanding complex systems. Farnham (United Kingdom): Ashgate; 2011.

42. Vincent C. Patient safety. 2nd edition. West Sussex (United K): John Wiley & Sons, Ltd; 2010.

43. Plsek PE, Greenhalgh T. Education and debate complexity science the challenge of complexity in health care. BMJ 2001;323:625–8.

44. Deutsch ES. More than complicated, healthcare delivery is complex, adaptive, and evolving. Pa Patient Saf Advis 2016;13(1):39–40.

45. Blanchard BS, Fabrycky WJ. Systems engineering and analysis. 5th edition. Boston: Prentice Hall; 2011.

46. Hollnagel E, Paries J, Woods DD, et al. Resilience engineering perspectives volume 3: resilience engineering in practice. Farnham (United Kingdom): Ashgate; 2011.

47. Woods DD. Essential characteristics of resilience. In: Hollnagel E, Woods DD, Leveson N, editors. Resilience engineering concepts and precepts. Hampshire (United Kingdom): Ashgate; 2006. p. 22.

48. Hollnagel E, Wears R, Braithwaite J. From safety-I to safety-II: a white paper. NHS England; 2015.

49. Vincent C, Amalberti R. Safer healthcare strategies for the real world. Cham (Switzerland): SpringerOpen; 2016.

50. Leveson N. A new accident model for engineering safer systems. Saf Sci 2004, 42:237–70.

51. Endsley MR. Toward a theory of situation awareness in dynamic systems. Hum Factors 1995;37(1):32–64.

52. Institute of Medicine Committee on Quality of Health Care in America. To err is human: building a safer health system. Washington, DC: National Academy Press; 1999.

53. Deutsch ES. That pesky human factor. Pa Patient Saf Advis 2016;13(2):79–80.

Anesthetic Considerations for Oral, Maxillofacial, and Neck Trauma

Jessica Lovich-Sapola, MD, MBA[a],*, Freedom Johnson, MD[b],
Charles E. Smith, MD[c]

KEYWORDS

- Maxillofacial trauma • Neck trauma • Airway • Hemorrhage • Anesthesia

KEY POINTS

- Airway injury is a major cause of early death in trauma patients.
- Bleeding, tissue derangement, and edema may make it difficult to access the airway, mask ventilate, or intubate the trachea.
- Facial trauma can be classified based on the anatomic location and displacement pattern of the facial bones: upper, mid and lower face, while neck trauma is classified by anatomic zones, which help predict organ injury, mortality, and ease of operative exposure.
- Signs and symptoms of laryngeal trauma include: subcutaneous emphysema, air escape, external bleeding or bruising, dyspnea, hypopnea, stridor, wheezing, cough, pain with phonation, dysphagia, hemoptysis, tracheal deviation, and nerve injury.
- The decisions regarding the approach and techniques used to support and maintain the patient's airway should be tailored to the patient's condition, clinical setting, injuries to the airway and other organs, and the available personnel, expertise, and equipment.

INTRODUCTION

Trauma is defined as physical damage to the body as a result of mechanical, chemical, thermal, electrical, or other energy that exceeds the tolerance of the body. Traumatic injuries kill more than 5 million people per year. In the United States, trauma (including unintentional injury, homicide, and suicide) was the third leading cause of death in

Disclosure: The authors have nothing to disclosure.
[a] Case Western Reserve University School of Medicine, MetroHealth Medical Center, Committee on Trauma and Emergency Preparedness, 2500 MetroHealth Drive, Cleveland, OH 44109, USA; [b] Department of Otolaryngology Head and Neck Surgery, Head and Neck Oncologic, Reconstructive and Cranial Base Surgery, Case Western Reserve University School of Medicine, MetroHealth Medical Center, 2500 MetroHealth Drive, Cleveland, OH 44109, USA; [c] Department of Anesthesiology, Case Western Reserve University School of Medicine, MetroHealth Medical Center, 2500 MetroHealth Drive, Cleveland, OH 44109, USA
* Corresponding author.
E-mail address: jlsapola@metrohealth.org

Otolaryngol Clin N Am 52 (2019) 1019–1035
https://doi.org/10.1016/j.otc.2019.08.004
0030-6665/19/© 2019 Elsevier Inc. All rights reserved.

2014 after heart disease and malignant neoplasms for people of all ages; it was also the leading cause of death in children and in adults up to 44 years of age.[1] Millions more suffer the physical and psychological consequences of trauma, which have an enormous impact on patients, their families, and society. In addition to death, the problem of nonfatal injury is staggering. In 2014, a total of 26.9 million people in the United States suffered nonfatal injuries requiring medical treatment. The total lifetime medical and work cost of injury and violence in the United States was $671 billion, of which $457 billion was the cost associated with nonfatal injuries.[1]

Blunt and penetrating trauma to the ear, nose, and throat (ENT) and related structures of the head and neck can be striking in presentation. Injuries may range from simple soft tissue wounds to complex injuries of the face, neck, and brain. The proximity of the cervical spine and airway further complicates anesthetic management of patients with otolaryngologic trauma. Functional, cosmetic, and social concerns are especially important. A multidisciplinary team approach is required. Control of the airway is the shared responsibility of the anesthesiologist and the ENT surgeon, and has the highest priority in the initial care of the injured patient. The perioperative management of the patient with otolaryngologic trauma is discussed.

OBJECTIVES

1. Review core principles in anesthesia for otolaryngology trauma, including management of the traumatized airway.
2. Discuss the anatomic considerations for otolaryngology trauma: maxillofacial, neck, and laryngotracheal.
3. Know the steps required to do a proper preoperative assessment and evaluation of a traumatized airway.
4. Formulate the anesthetic plan for patients undergoing surgery for otolaryngology trauma.

EPIDEMIOLOGY AND MECHANISM OF INJURY

Airway injury is a major cause of early death in trauma patients.[2] Although the overall incidence of airway injury in a trauma is low (<1%), the mortality due to traumatic airway injuries is high, in part because of associated trauma to other body systems, such as neurologic, thoracic, abdominal, and skeletal systems.[2] Because airway injuries are an infrequent occurrence, it can be difficult to maintain well-developed assessment and management skills, resulting in staff being less prepared to deal with such situations.[2] Vehicular trauma is the primary cause of maxillofacial trauma, followed by assault, sports injuries, falls, and civilian warfare.[3] Maxillofacial injuries often occur in the setting of polytrauma and require a coordinated approach from multiple physician specialties, including emergency physicians, anesthesiologists, otolaryngology specialists, maxillofacial/plastic and reconstructive surgeons, orthopedists, ophthalmologists, and neurosurgeons.[3] According to the Advanced Trauma Life Support (ATLS) handbook, the loss of an airway kills faster than the loss of the ability to breathe or hemorrhagic shock, because acute airway obstruction and respiratory arrest cause hypoxic brain injury and death.[3]

MECHANISMS OF INJURY

Common mechanisms of airway trauma include[4]:

- Penetrating injury: gunshot or knife wounds
- Blunt trauma: motor vehicle collisions, falls, hanging, or violent crime

- Blast injury
- Burns: chemical, electrical or flame

Penetrating injury may result in the loss of anatomic landmarks secondary to broken bones and teeth.[4] Bleeding, tissue derangement, and edema may make it difficult to access the airway, mask ventilate, or intubate the trachea.[4] Patients may develop rapid airway obstruction and neurovascular compromise[5] (**Figs. 1–3**).

Blunt trauma usually results in less soft tissue damage and less obliteration of facial structures than penetrating trauma.[4,5] Facial fractures from blunt trauma result in airway compromise because of either posterior displacement of the midface structures into the oropharynx, retropulsion of the tongue and soft tissue with resultant airway obstruction owing to loss of mandibular bony integrity, and/or obstruction a result of severe swelling and hemorrhage.[5]

Blast injuries have 3 mechanisms of injury[5]:

- Primary: mass movement of air
  - Damage to maxillofacial area, sinuses, tympanic membrane, lungs
- Secondary: flying debris
  - Causes most casualties during an explosion
- Tertiary: victims are thrown
  - Multiple injuries
  - Gross contamination of wounds

Burns from chemicals, electricity, or flame may cause severe obliteration of the airway secondary to the associated soft tissue edema and friability.[4,5] Immediate airway management is often required before the airway is compromised by the ongoing edema, especially in patients with stridor and respiratory distress.[5]

Signs of smoke exposure and inhalational injury include[6]:

- Soot in the nares
- Singed facial hair
- Carbonaceous sputum
- Increased respiratory rate, dyspnea, use of accessory muscles, progressive hoarseness, stridor

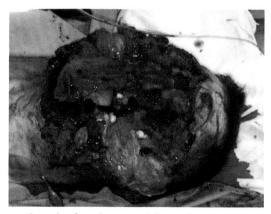

Fig. 1. Gunshot wound to the face (young adult man). On emergency medical services arrival patient was breathing spontaneously and attempting to speak. The airway was secured in the field with orotracheal intubation. (*Courtesy of* F. Johnson, MD, FACS, Cleveland, OH.)

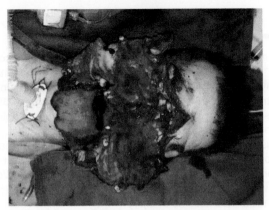

Fig. 2. Man from **Fig. 1**. Gunshot wound to the face, after tracheostomy and surgical positioning of tissue. (*Courtesy of* F. Johnson, MD, FACS, Cleveland, OH.)

- Increased secretions
- Dysphagia
- Elevated carbon monoxide level greater than 15%
- Visible airway edema

ANATOMIC CONSIDERATIONS

The facial skeleton is composed of many bones that interdigitate with each other at suture lines.[7] In the setting of trauma, these suture lines may act as crumple zones

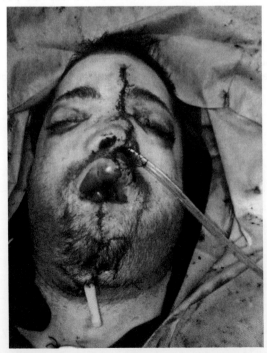

Fig. 3. Male gunshot wound from **Figs. 1** and **2** after initial surgical repair. (*Courtesy of* F. Johnson, MD, FACS, Cleveland, OH.)

to evenly distribute the energy transferred to the face, which may provide a protective advantage by minimizing damage to the skull and brain.[7] As a result of the overall bony anatomy, facial fractures tend to occur at characteristic points where the bones are weakest.[7] Although this may protect the brain, the airway is often compromised. In addition to direct physical damage, in many trauma situations airway instability can be exacerbated by diminished level of consciousness, alcohol and/or drug intoxication, altered laryngeal reflexes, and increased risk of aspiration.[8] Traumatic airway injuries can be divided into 3 types: maxillofacial, neck, and laryngotracheal injuries[2] (**Figs. 4** and **5**).

Maxillofacial Trauma

Facial trauma can be classified based on the anatomic location and displacement pattern of the facial bones.[4] The face is divided into equal thirds[3,7]:

- Upper face: hairline to glabella
  - Frontal bone
  - Frontal sinuses
  - Craniofacial Junction
- Midface: glabella to columella (This area is considered the "crumple zone" to protect the brain.)
  - Maxilla
  - Nasal bones
  - Nasoethmoidal complex

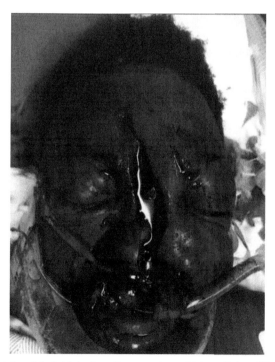

Fig. 4. Man with trilevel facial injuries after a motor vehicle collision. (*Courtesy of* F. Johnson, MD, FACS, Cleveland, OH.)

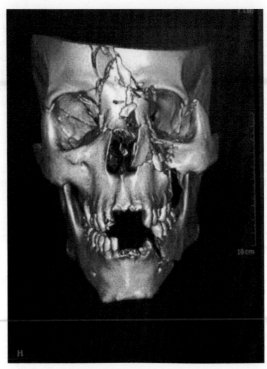

Fig. 5. 3D computed tomography scan of patient in **Fig. 4** showing trilevel facial fractures including comminuted fronto-ethmodial-orbital, left zygomaticomaxillary complex, and left mandibular fractures. Patient had CSF leak owing to involvement of the anterior cranial fossa. (*Courtesy of* F. Johnson, MD, FACS, Cleveland, OH.)

- ○ Zygomaticomaxillary complex
- ○ Orbital floor/eyes
- • Lower face
- ○ Dentoalveolar
- ○ Mandible

Upper face

Isolated upper face fractures have a limited direct impact on airway but are often associated with intracranial and cervical spine injuries.

Midface

Midface fractures can lead to airway edema and airway compromise primarily through loss of the nasal/nasopharyngeal airway.[4] They are also associated with intracranial and cervical spine injuries.[4] These injuries may result in a significant amount of blood being swallowed and therefore can result in vomiting and aspiration.[4]

Maxillary fractures are classified also into 3 areas[2–4]:

- • Le Fort I: horizontal fracture that separates the tooth-bearing part of the maxilla and the hard palate from the rest of the maxilla
- ○ Loose dentition, bleeding, and difficult mask ventilation are concerns for the airway

- Le Fort II: pyramid-shaped fracture that separates the maxilla and nose from the upper lateral midface and zygoma
  - Concern is for possible associated skull base fracture and leakage of cerebrospinal fluid (CSF)
    - Mask ventilation may lead to pneumocephalus
  - Epistaxis and facial swelling can make mask ventilation and visualization of the airway difficult during laryngoscopy (conventional/video) or flexible bronchoscopy
- Le Fort III: separation of all facial bones from the cranial base, the midface is typically separated and displace posteriorly
  - Fracture of the zygoma, maxilla, and nasal bones
  - Concern is for possible associated skull base fracture and leakage of CSF
  - Blind nasotracheal intubation or nasogastric tube placement is avoided secondary to the risk of intracranial penetration of the tube
  - Face mask ventilation is often difficult secondary to facial edema, CSF leak, and epistaxis
  - Associated with head and cervical spine injuries

Zygomatic arch fractures may result in limited jaw opening due to mechanical restriction from bony impingement on the mandibular coronoid process, which can affect the ability to orotracheally intubate the patient.[4] These fractures are often associated with orbital and eye injury.[2] Patients may present with vision loss or changes, traumatic mydriasis, and/or increased intraocular pressure.[2]

Lower face

Dental injuries can result in avulsed and/or fractured teeth, tongue laceration, soft tissue swelling, and oral cavity hemorrhage.[2] It is important that each tooth a patient had before his/her injury is accounted for.[9] A radiographic examination should be performed to look for lost teeth to verify that they are not in the tracheobronchial tree or gastrointestinal tract.[9]

The mandible is the second-most commonly fractured bone of the face after the nose.[9] The mandibular ring rarely breaks in only one place; therefore, mandible fractures often occur in 2 or more places owing to its "U" shape.[4,7] Bilateral (bucket handle) fractures of the anterior mandible are associated with loss of tongue support and may result in airway obstruction from posterior displacement of the tongue.[2,4] This obstruction can be treated with upright positioning of the patient if they are not at risk of cervical spinal cord injury, or by manual anterior displacement of the tongue/mandible.[2] It is important to remember that limited mouth opening from a mandible fracture may be because of mechanical obstruction (displaced condylar fracture fragment, concomitant depressed zygomatic arch fracture) and not pain or trismus, and therefore may not improve after the induction of anesthesia and neuromuscular blockade.[2,4]

Neck Trauma

Neck trauma is classified by anatomic zones, which help predict organ injury, mortality, and ease of operative exposure.[10]

- Zone I comprises the thoracic inlet, which is bound inferiorly by the sternal notch and superiorly by the cricoid cartilage. Structures include the great vessels of the thoracic inlet and the cervical esophagus. Proximal vascular control in this zone is difficult, mandating adequate intravenous access and access to blood and blood products (massive transfusion protocol) and arterial line monitoring.

- Zone II is from the cricoid cartilage to the angle of the mandible. Proximal and distal vascular control are easier to obtain than in zone I injuries (**Fig. 6**).
- Zone III injuries extend from the angle of the mandible to skull base. As with zone I injuries, distal control of bleeding is more difficult.

Neck wounds may extend downward and enter the chest cavity with resultant massive bleeding, pneumothorax, shock, and difficult ventilation. Emergent tube thoracostomy may be necessary. While assessing a patient for significant neck injury, the physician should look for active external bleeding from a wound, dysphagia, stridor, subcutaneous emphysema (possibly because of the disruption of the larynx or trachea), expanding hematoma, sucking neck wound, or neurologic deficit a result of a spinal cord or brachial plexus injury.[2] Preoperative angiography or computed tomography (CT) angiography is often of benefit. Early deaths are associated with asphyxia from airway compromise or arterial hypotension.[2] The airway may be compressed by tissue disruption, edema, or hematoma.[2]

Any patient with a penetrating neck wound and airway compromise should undergo emergent airway control. Endotracheal intubation should be done by experienced personnel, and physicians must be available to perform a surgical airway should tracheal intubation be unsuccessful. After securing the airway, the patient should undergo formal neck exploration. Neck wounds should never be probed or explored outside of the operating room because of the risk of dislodging a thrombus and resultant uncontrolled hemorrhage.[2]

Laryngotracheal Trauma

Signs and symptoms of laryngeal trauma include: subcutaneous emphysema, air escape, external bleeding or bruising, dyspnea, hypopnea, stridor, wheezing, cough, pain with phonation, dysphagia, hemoptysis, tracheal deviation, and nerve injury.[2] These injuries can be confirmed with bedside flexible laryngoscopy, bronchoscopy, or CT scan.[2] Laryngotracheal injury is often associated with injuries to the cervical spine, skull base, cervicothoracic vasculature, and esophagus.[2]

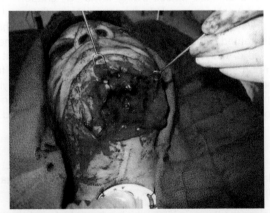

Fig. 6. Submental gunshot wound (zone 2 of the neck). Entry wound at submental region, exit at left naso-orbital region. Patient presented awake, alert, oriented and breathing spontaneously. The airway was secured with planned orotracheal intubation with rapid sequence induction after discussing with patient. (*Courtesy of* F. Johnson, MD, FACS, Cleveland, OH.)

One specific injury that requires special attention is laryngo-tracheal separation.[2] In this situation, insertion of an endotracheal tube may worsen the separation and convert a tenuous airway into a lost airway.[2] This is most common in deceleration trauma causing flexion-extension of the neck and resulting in a shearing-off of the trachea at the cricoid and/or carina because they are anchored to other anatomic structures.[2] For patients with airway disruption, the goal is to pass the endotracheal tube across the injured area without causing further disruption or to bypass the injury by inserting the tube distal to the injury using a surgical approach.[2]

Blunt trauma may result in a crushing or transection of the laryngeal cartilages and/ or tracheal rings by compression against the cervical spine.[2] In cases of a complete transection, the cervical trachea may retract into the mediastinum.[2]

PREOPERATIVE ASSESSMENT AND EVALUATION OF THE TRAUMATIZED AIRWAY

Before arrival, the prehospital personnel should communicate the patient's mechanism of injury, age, Glasgow Coma Scale (GCS), vital signs, and anticipated time of arrival[11] (**Table 1**). While the focus should be on the mechanism and extent of the injury, it is important to know any other pertinent medical history, including anticoagulation medications that may lead to excessive hemorrhage[4] (**Box 1**).

ATLS stresses the importance of remembering to treat the greatest threat first, and that a detailed history is not as important as treating significant acute injuries.[2] If oxygenation and ventilation can be maintained in the prehospital setting, then a definitive airway should not be placed, and the attempt may in fact be detrimental.[2] Once the patient arrives at the hospital, radiologic findings such as chest radiographs, spine evaluations, ultrasound, and head/maxillofacial CT may be useful to provide comprehensive information about the structures around the airway and any airway compromise.[2,4]

Table 1
Glasgow Coma Scale score

		Score
Best eye response	Spontaneous	4
	To speech	3
	To pain	2
	None	1
Best verbal response	Oriented	5
	Disoriented	4
	Inappropriate words	3
	Incomprehensible sounds	2
	None	1
Best motor response	Obeys verbal orders	6
	Localize pain	5
	Flexion (withdrawal) to pain	4
	Flexion (decortication) to pain	3
	Extension (decerebration) to pain	2
	None (flaccid)	1

Total Glasgow Coma Scale score (range 3–15) is summation of best eye + verbal + motor response scores. Traumatic brain injury is classified severe if GCS score is ≤8 and is associated with higher morbidity and mortality. It is classified moderate if GCS score is 9 to 12 and mild if the GCS score 13 to 15.

Modified from Dagal A and Lam AM. Head trauma: anesthetic considerations and management. In Smith CE, ed. Trauma Anesthesia 2nd ed. New York, NY: Cambridge University Press; 2015: 364-379; with permission.

Box 1
Preoperative anesthetic assessment checklist for trauma

1. Airway and cervical spine stability

2. Adequacy of oxygenation and ventilation

3. Blood pressure, heart rate, and rhythm

4. Baseline neurologic status

5. Associated injuries

6. Available medical, surgical, and anesthetic history, and allergies

7. Baseline imaging studies (CXR, CT scans, FAST examination)

8. Current medications including anticoagulant/antiplatelet use (eg, direct factor Xa inhibitors, direct thrombin inhibitors, clopidogrel, aspirin, or warfarin) and herbal supplements

9. Relevant laboratory data (eg, hematocrit, coagulation profile, blood gas, glucose, electrolytes)

10. Planning of the postoperative management and discharge destination (eg, PACU, ICU)

Abbreviations: CT, computed tomography; CXR, chest x-ray (radiograph); FAST, focused assessment with sonography in trauma; ICU, intensive care unit; PACU, postanesthesia care unit.
    Modified from Werner S. Trauma in the prehospital environment and the emergency department. In Smith CE, ed. Trauma Anesthesia 2nd ed. New York, NY: Cambridge University Press; 2015. 6-26, with permission.

Neurologic assessments[2,4]:

- Altered level of consciousness
  ○ GCS less than 9 results in loss of the protective airway reflexes
  ○ Shock
  ○ Brain injury
  ○ Intoxication (alcohol, other drugs)
- Paralysis
- Pupillary size
- Clinical signs of elevated intracranial pressure: hypertension, bradycardia, and irregular breathing

Airway assessment should be as complete as possible, but done quickly, because the rapid development of facial edema or hematoma may lead to airway obstruction.[2,4] Airway compromise secondary to edema and hematoma may evolve over time; therefore, the patient should be reevaluated frequently for the first few hours.[2]
Airway evaluation[2,4,8]:

- Continuous oxygen saturation monitoring
- Facial deformities
  ○ Mandible fractures leading to loss of tongue support
  ○ Posterior displacement of the midface structures into the oropharynx
- Swelling of soft tissues
  ○ Face, tongue, or neck
  ○ Inability to swallow
  ○ Hematoma
- Retropharyngeal hematoma from a cervical spine injury
  ○ Risk of airway collapse
  ○ Impairs visualization of the larynx during intubation

- Neck motion
  - Associated spine injury
- Dental injury
- Nasal patency
- Mouth opening
- Mallampati score
- Palpation of the larynx and trachea for deviation or collapse
- Impending respiratory compromise
  - Cyanosis
  - Dysphonia
  - Inspiratory or biphasic stridor
  - Agitation
  - Dyspnea
  - Accessory muscle use
  - Requests to sit up or lean forward
- Foreign body
  - Blood
  - Secretions
  - Teeth/dentures
  - Food
  - Vomit

ANESTHETIC MANAGEMENT OF THE AIRWAY

Airway management for the trauma patient may occur in a variety of settings: emergency room, operating room, radiology suite, or intensive care unit. Management may vary in the severity or mechanism of the airway injury.[11] The tools and algorithms to manage the airway in a trauma patient are like those used in a nonemergency situation.[11] However, the important difference is that the awakening of a patient if there is a failed intubation is typically not an option.[11]

Initial assessment of the patient's ventilatory status should include a simple question such as "What is your name?"[11] An appropriate response shows intact ventilation, patent airway, and appropriate circulatory perfusion to the brain.[2,11] If breathing is compromised, the goal is to place a cuffed endotracheal tube below the level of the vocal cords.[11]

ATLS has definitive indications for securing an airway, including the need for oxygenation or ventilation (cardiac arrest, shock, inadequate respiratory effort, hypoxia, severe agitation, massive blood loss, GCS $\leq$8, and/or apnea) or the need for airway protection (severe maxillofacial fractures, risk of airway obstruction, risk of aspiration, or unconsciousness).[2,11] Esophageal injury occurs in up to 10% of patients with laryngotracheal trauma. These patients also require intubation.[2] Early airway control is also recommended for hematomas or exposure to chemical, biological, or inhalation agents, including smoke and burns that can cause increasing mucosal edema.[2,6]

Clinicians must always ensure the immediate availability of adequate airway equipment including[4,12]:

- Protective gear
- Oxygen
- Masks of multiple sizes
- Bag-mask ventilation device capable of delivering positive-pressure ventilation
- High volume suction
- Laryngoscope blades, video-assisted intubating devices, flexible bronchoscope

- Nasal and oral airways
- Endotracheal tubes, multiple sizes
- Endotracheal tube stylets
- Gum-elastic bougie (tracheal tube introducer)
- Laryngeal mask airway or a laryngeal tube airway
- Cricothyroidotomy kit
- Intravenous setup
- Induction and resuscitation medications
- Medications to anesthetize the airway
- American Society of Anesthesiologists (ASA) standard monitors including an instrument to measure end-tidal CO_2

Emergency airway medications should include an induction agent such as propofol, etomidate, or ketamine, and a fast-acting paralytic such as succinylcholine or rocuronium.[11] Propofol can be used but may cause profound hypotension in hypovolemic patients.[11] Etomidate causes less hemodynamic changes than propofol but is associated with adrenal suppression.[11] Ketamine may cause tachycardia and hypertension secondary to the endogenous catecholamine release, which may be helpful in the trauma setting.[11] All trauma patients are considered as "full-stomach."[3] A rapid sequence induction (RSI) and intubation with or without cricoid pressure is typically the technique of choice in patients with adequate mouth opening.[4]

Cricoid pressure is the technique by which pressure is applied to the cricoid cartilage at the neck to potentially occlude the esophagus that passes behind it and help reduce the risk of regurgitation.[12] Although the principle seems logical, there is no evidence that it actually works to reduce aspiration risk. Cricoid pressure requires 20 to 30 N of force and is therefore often contraindicated in the presence of airway injury.[12] RSI and intubation is the most common method for securing a definitive airway in a trauma patient.[11] It is essential to be prepared to suction and manually clear the airway of any debris during the intubation.[2]

Trauma patients may present unexpected challenges when securing the airway.[11] Preoxygenation with 100% oxygen for 3 to 5 minutes is important before any intubation attempts because of the increased risk of poor patient cooperation or patient injury that may impose a time constraint while securing the airway.[2,11] This preoxygenation increases the duration of adequate oxygenation during the period of postinduction apnea.[12] Oxygen (100%) should be applied to any trauma patient as soon as they are encountered in the field or trauma bay.[12] It should be recognized that the ability to preoxygenate may be difficult or impossible secondary to a difficult mask seal, and that positive pressure mask ventilation may result in worsening of facial fractures and increased airway compression.[2,4]

Often, the status of the cervical spine is unknown, and care should be taken to prevent inadvertent neurologic injury. The incidence of cervical spine injury in the adult population after a blunt trauma is only about 1% to 3%.[13] When tracheal intubation is required in a cooperative patient with a high suspicion for cervical spine injury, the airway can be secured using an awake technique with topical anesthesia and maintenance of spontaneous ventilation.[2,11] If the patient is cooperative, a fiberoptic bronchoscope with minimal neck movement is a safe approach.[11] Often, the cervical collar can remain in place. The benefit of an awake intubation is that it allows for a neurologic assessment immediately after intubation.[11] One caveat in an airway trauma patient is that blood, secretions, or emesis can make visualization with the fiberoptic scope difficult or impossible.[4,11] More often than not, the trauma patient cannot tolerate an awake intubation because of shock, altered mentation, and other factors.

In these situations, RSI may be done, and restriction of spinal motion can be achieved using manual in-line stabilization (MILS) of the neck during the RSI.[11] This technique requires an additional person to maintain MILS so that spinal motion can be minimized during placement of the endotracheal tube.[2] The anterior portion of the cervical collar should be removed during an RSI with MILS to facilitate mouth opening.[11] MILS can be modified if it is preventing intubation.[11]

The ASA has a well-defined algorithm for patients with a difficult airway.[11] There are a few modifications for trauma patients.[11]

- In a controlled setting, an expected difficult intubation patient should have an awake intubation. In a trauma, if the patient is unstable or uncooperative, induction of general anesthesia may be required even for patients with an expected difficult airway.
- If noninvasive measures to secure the airway are unsuccessful, a surgical airway may be required if the emergency does not allow time to wake the patient or delay the surgery.

Video laryngoscopy has become the most common first-line rescue airway device in a trauma setting because of the improved first-pass success rate and improved view of the glottis when compared with direct laryngoscopy.[11] This does not imply that direct laryngoscopy is not effective; indeed, conventional laryngoscopy may be superior to video laryngoscopy in certain situations such as poor opening of the mouth and blood or emesis in the airway.[11]

A supraglottic device, such as a laryngeal mask airway or a laryngeal tube airway, is used in the ASA difficult airway algorithm and ATLS in the case of "cannot intubate, cannot ventilate."[11] Once the laryngeal mask airway is in place, an airway exchange catheter can be used to facilitate exchange with an endotracheal tube. Alternatively, an endotracheal tube can be placed although the supraglottic device using a fiberoptic scope.[11] It is important to remember that a supraglottic device is not a definitive airway and does not protect the patient from aspiration of upper airway material.[4]

Intubating the trachea with a lighted stylet (light wand) or a retrograde wire technique are often contraindicated in an airway trauma patient because these blind techniques can lead to worsening of laryngeal injuries.[4] Nasal airways and blind nasotracheal intubation should also be avoided if there is any concern of skull base fracture or nasal fracture.[2]

A surgical airway may be the definitive first choice to secure the airway in an otherwise cooperative patient with a difficult airway who is not in significant respiratory distress.[4] The incidence of an emergency surgical airway in a trauma patient is very low (0.3%).[11] Once general anesthesia is induced, the team must be prepared to proceed with surgical interventions if the noninvasive airway technique is not successful.[11] A cricothyroidotomy is the most common method to surgically establish an emergency airway.[11] The open technique is the fastest method and has been shown to be safe and efficient even when placed by less experienced providers.[11] A tracheotomy is not the most rapid method to obtain a surgical airway but does result in fewer long-term complications.[11] However, the increased time and increased risk of bleeding often outweigh these benefits in an emergency setting.[11]

Securing the airway of a patient with a penetrating neck injury has its own challenges.[11] The injury may interfere with successful intubation or the intubation itself may cause a worsening of the patient's injury.[11] Blind intubation methods should be avoided. Awake fiberoptic or RSI fiberoptic intubation are often the preferred intubation methods in these situations. Other methods used are RSI with direct laryngoscopy or video laryngoscopy, and finally a surgical airway if the above methods fail.[11] Once the airway is secured, the cuff of the endotracheal tube must be positioned below the injury to prevent air leak.[11] If the patient has an overt airway injury that opens to the skin, intubation can be done through the open wound.[11]

In select cases, submental intubation may be used to avoid a tracheostomy and nasal intubation.[3] With submental intubation, the patient's trachea is first intubated orally, often with an armored, reinforced tube.[13] A 2-cm incision is made halfway between the chin and angle of the mandible, and blunt dissection is performed to the oral floor.[3] The endotracheal tube is then pulled through this canal and connected to the ventilator.[3] The tube is then sutured to the skin.[13] The benefit of this technique is that the operating field is clear of the endotracheal tube. Submental intubation can be maintained for up to 48 hours; after 48 hours, there is an increased risk of infection.[3]

Retromolar intubation may be used after a standard oral intubation. The endotracheal tube is moved to the space posterior to the last molar and anterior to the ascending mandibular ramus, or the missing tooth space.[5] This method is used for patients who need simultaneous nasal surgery and restoration of dental occlusion.[5] A reinforced endotracheal tube is advised to avoid kinking. The technique is noninvasive, fast, and easy.[5]

BLEEDING

Maxillofacial injuries rarely bleed enough to cause hemorrhagic shock.[3,4] Most injuries result in slow venous bleeding from the nose or mouth that can be controlled.[4] Blood may accumulate in the oropharynx and can lead to obstruction and impaired visualization of the airway.[2,4] The supine position of the facial trauma patient increases the risk of swallowing the blood with subsequent aspiration.[2,4] Damage control maneuvers to stop the bleeding can be accomplished through nasal/oral gauze pressure packing, ligation, nasal balloon tamponade, and/or rapid manual fracture reduction and stabilization of displaced bone fragments.[2–4,8] Angiographic trans-arterial embolization or surgical intervention may be required to stop some bleeds.[2,4,8] Selective embolization is not favored because of its high complication risk and should only be used as a last resort.[8] These complications include: 7th nerve palsy, trismus, necrosis of the tongue, blindness, migration of emboli, and stroke.[8] Emergency evacuation of the hematoma may be required to prevent worsening airway obstruction.[7]

ELECTIVE VERSUS EMERGENCY SURGERY

The timing of the surgical repair of a facial trauma depends on the extent and severity of the injuries.[4] Life-, sight-, or limb-threatening injuries should be treated first.[5] Contaminated facial wounds require surgery within a few hours if the patient is otherwise stable.[5] Definitive repairs may be delayed until the patient is stable, pertinent evaluations and studies are completed, and the facial edema has resolved.[4]

The repairs of traumatic facial injuries often require multiple surgeries.[5]

1. Debridement and initial stabilization of the fractures
2. Hard tissue reconstruction
3. Rehabilitation and secondary closure of residual deformities

Mandible fractures are usually repaired at 24 to 48 hours and other fractures by 7 to 10 days.[4,9] After 10 to 14 days the injury becomes more difficult to treat and reduce correctly.[4,9] Although the timing may differ, the goal is always function and cosmetic restoration and prevention of complications such as: malunion, CSF leak, globe injury, extraocular muscle entrapment, brain abscess, osteomyelitis, and sinusitis.[9]

INTRAOPERATIVE ANESTHETIC CONSIDERATIONS

Considerations include: length of surgery, airway issues, estimated blood loss, hemodynamic status, and requirements for postoperative ventilation.[4] Constant communication between the anesthesia and surgical teams about the plan and goals is of utmost importance for achieving the best outcome.[4] Induction of anesthesia should be free of wide variations in blood pressure, which could lead to excessive bleeding or impair perfusion for vital organs.[4] The clinician should always be mindful of possible associated intracranial injuries with all facial trauma patients[4] (**Table 2**).

Maintenance of anesthesia can be provided with inhalational or total intravenous anesthetics.[4] Dexmedetomidine may be a useful adjunct to provide sedation

Table 2
Goals of general anesthesia for trauma

Goal	Techniques
Reestablish and maintain normal hemodynamics	1. For hypotension, fluids first, then vasopressors 2. Frequent evaluation of acid-base status, hematocrit, urinary output 3. Titration of additional anesthetics if satisfactory blood pressure 4. Monitor pulse pressure and systolic pressure variation. Administer fluid boluses as indicated
Maximize surgical exposure and minimize edema	1. Limit fluids according to needs 2. Limit blood loss by allowing anesthetic catch-up 3. Optimize neuromuscular blockade 4. Nasogastric or orogastric tube to decompress bowel 5. Avoid nitrous oxide
Limit hypothermia	1. Monitor core temperature 2. Warm intravenous fluids and blood 3. Keep patient covered 4. Warm the operating room (>28°C) 5. Apply convective warming blanket
Help limit blood loss and coagulopathy	1. Encourage the surgeon to stop and pack if blood loss is excessive (damage control) 2. Frequently monitor hematocrit, ionized Ca, coagulation studies 3. Provide calcium for large citrated product administration 4. Administer plasma, platelets, cryoprecipitate, fibrinogen, factor concentrates including prothrombin complex concentrate as clinically indicated or according to point of care coagulation tests (ROTEM, TEG)
Limit complications to other systems	1. Maintain cerebral perfusion pressure >70 mm Hg if associated head injury 2. Monitor peak airway pressures and tidal volumes. Tidal volumes 5–6 ml/kg ideal body weight, Peak + plateau pressures <30 mm H_2O, positive end-expiratory pressure as needed to maintain Pao_2 >60 mm Hg, Permissive hypercapnia if no head injury 3. Be vigilant for pneumothorax 4. Measure urine output 5. Monitor peripheral pulses

Modified from Bassett M and Smith CE. General Anesthesia for Trauma. In Varon AJ and Smith CE, ed. Essentials of Trauma Anesthesia 2nd ed. New York, NY: Cambridge University Press; 2018: 82-101; with permission.

without risk of respiratory depression. An arterial line is indicated for surgeries requiring controlled hypotension to help minimize surgical bleeding. Intraoperative assessment of nerve function may be required by the surgical team; if so, neuromuscular blockade should be avoided in these cases.[4] Vecuronium and rocuronium neuromuscular block can be reversed with sugammadex, if required. Fluid management should be targeted to ensure adequate blood and fluid replacement and to maintain hemodynamic normality.[4] Static and dynamic hemodynamic parameters for prediction of fluid responsiveness are generally employed. Pulse pressure variation, stroke volume variation, and systolic pressure variation can be obtained using arterial line monitoring and pulse contour analysis. The anesthesia team should be prepared for surgical blood loss with large-bore intravenous catheters, fluid replacement, and proper blood sampling.[7] Atropine should be available in the case of oculo-cardiac reflex and reflex bradycardia from the manipulation of the midface.[7]

Emergence and extubation must be planned with the surgical team.[4] These patients are often considered at high risk of extubation.[3] The degree of airway edema can continue to worsen during the first 48 hours after the injury.[7] Patients should not be extubated until they are fully awake, airway reflexes return, and are obeying commands.[3] Emergency intubation medications and airway equipment should be available at extubation.[7] Consideration may be given to the placement of an airway exchange catheter that is left in place after extubation. Reintubation can then be performed through this catheter if needed.[13] The surgical team should remain at the bedside until after the extubation.[7] If the patient's trachea is extubated in the operating room, the patient should be observed closely in a high observation unit with continuous pulse oximetry in the immediate postoperative period.[7,13]

POSTOPERATIVE CONSIDERATIONS

Judicious use of postoperative nausea and vomiting prophylaxis is recommended. Also, effective multimodal pain control should be supplied, using local anesthetic, NSAIDS, acetaminophen, and opioids.[3,7] Intravenous dexamethasone should be given to decrease the swelling, and prophylactic antibiotics given if the wound is grossly contaminated, it is open to the oral cavity, cartilage is exposed, or the wound has been devascularized.[7]

Patients with maxillomandibular fixation should have wire cutters or scissors for elastic bands at their bedside at all times in case of vomiting or airway obstruction.[4,7]

Patients with risk of further swelling or bleeding, particularly Le Fort II and III fractures, require postoperative observation in an intensive care setting for the first 12 to 24 hours.[4]

SUMMARY

Otolaryngology trauma patient management is complex and there is a lack of evidence-based approaches regarding the best practice for management of the patient's airway. The usual techniques of airway, breathing, and circulation management need to be tailored to the patient's injuries and comorbidities. A multidisciplinary approach is required for optimal outcomes. Airway control is the prime concern. Decisions regarding the approach and techniques used to support and maintain the patient's airway should be based on the patient's condition, clinical setting, injuries to the airway and other organs, and the available personnel, expertise, and equipment.

REFERENCES

1. Como JJ, Smith CE. Trauma epidemiology, mechanisms of injury, and prehospital care. In: Varon AJ, Smith CE, editors. Essentials of trauma anesthesia. 2nd edition. New York: Cambridge University Press; 2018. p. 1–15.
2. Jain U, McCunn M, Smith CE, et al. Management of the traumatized airway. Anesthesiology 2016;124(1):199–206.
3. Singh S, Kumar S, Kumar K, et al. Anesthetic challenges and management of maxillofacial trauma. J Anesth Surg 2017;4(2):134–40.
4. Gollapudy S, Kaslow O. Anesthetic considerations for ocular and maxillofacial trauma. In: Varon AJ, Smith CE, editors. Essentials of trauma anesthesia. 2nd edition. New York: Cambridge University Press; 2018. p. 200–11.
5. Kaslow O, Holak EJ. Anesthesia for oral and maxillofacial trauma. In: Smith CE, editor. Trauma anesthesia. 2nd edition. New York: Cambridge University Press; 2015. p. 426–36.
6. Lovich-Sapola JA. Anesthesia for burns. In: Smith CE, editor. Trauma anesthesia. 2nd edition. New York: Cambridge University Press; 2015. p. 666–88.
7. Morosan M, Parbhoo A, Curry N. Anaesthesia and common oral and maxillafacial emergencies. Cont Educ Anaesth Crit Care Pain 2012;12(5):257–62.
8. Jose A, Nagori SA, Agarwal B, et al. Management of maxillofacial trauma in emergency: An update of challenges and controversies. J Emerg Trauma Shock 2016; 9(2):73–80.
9. Guglielmi M, Shaikh R, Parekh KP, et al. Oral and maxillofacial trauma: surgical considerations. In: Smith CE, editor. Trauma anesthesia. 2nd edition. New York: Cambridge University Press; 2015. p. 412–25.
10. Low GM, Inaba K, Chouliaras K, et al. The use of the anatomic 'zones' of the neck in the assessment of penetrating neck injury. Am Surg 2014;80(10):970–4.
11. Diez C, Varon AAJ. Airway management. In: Varon AJ, Smith CE, editors. Essentials of trauma anesthesia. 2nd edition. New York: Cambridge University Press; 2018. p. 29–43.
12. O'Brien O, Wilson W. Trauma airway management. In: Smith CE, editor. Trauma anesthesia. 2nd edition. New York: Cambridge University Press; 2015. p. 27–64.
13. Kellman RM, Losquadro WD. Comprehensive airway management of patients with maxillofacial trauma. Craniomaxillofac Trauma Reconstr 2008;1(1):39–47.

Anesthesia in Diagnostic and Therapeutic Pediatric Bronchoscopy

Aldo V. Londino III, MD[a], Narasimhan Jagannathan, MD, MBA[b],*

KEYWORDS

- Rigid bronchoscopy • Flexible bronchoscopy
- Therapeutic & diagnostic airway endoscopy
- Airway management during airway endoscopy • Airway foreign body

KEY POINTS

- Airway endoscopy (rigid and flexible bronchoscopy) is an important procedure that allows for visualization of the trachea and bronchi as well as treatment of a variety of airway disorders for diagnostic and therapeutic interventions.
- There must be excellent communication between the anesthesiologist and the endoscopist to ensure that adequate oxygenation and ventilation is maintained via the shared airway.
- Various anesthetic and airway management techniques can be used for airway management in pediatric foreign-body aspiration.

INTRODUCTION

Airway bronchoscopy is an important procedure that allows for visualization of the trachea and bronchi as well as treatment of a variety of airway disorders in the pediatric patient population. The last 2 centuries have witnessed significant advances in bronchoscopy with the development of the rigid endoscope, the glass-rod telescope, high-definition cameras, and advanced anesthetic techniques. The successful execution of these procedures relies on a skilled surgeon, an experienced anesthesiologist, an attentive support staff, and good communication and coordination among all team members. This article highlights the indications, techniques, and complications encountered during pediatric bronchoscopy, with particular focus on anesthetic management of the pediatric airway.

[a] The Mount Sinai Hospital, One Gustave L. Levy Place, New York, NY 10029, USA; [b] Academic Affairs, Pediatric Anesthesia Research, Department of Pediatric Anesthesiology, Northwestern University Feinberg School of Medicine, Ann & Robert H. Lurie Children's Hospital of Chicago, 225 East Chicago Avenue, Chicago, IL 60611, USA
* Corresponding author.
E-mail address: njagannathan@luriechildrens.org

Otolaryngol Clin N Am 52 (2019) 1037–1048
https://doi.org/10.1016/j.otc.2019.08.005
0030-6665/19/© 2019 Elsevier Inc. All rights reserved.

CASE PRESENTATION: FOREIGN-BODY ASPIRATION

A toddler is brought into the emergency room after a witnessed choking spell while eating peanuts. He has recovered well; however, since the incident the child has developed a persistent cough with an increased work of breathing and stridor. The child presents with a respiratory rate of 40/min, a heart rate of 140 beats/min, and an oxygen saturation of 92% on room air. Auscultation of the lungs reveals coarse breath sounds and wheezing in the right lung base. The child has evidence of right-sided air trapping on plain film of the chest. The pediatric pulmonary, otolaryngology, and anesthesiology teams are consulted.

Historically, children with the diagnosis of an airway foreign body could expect a difficult clinical course with a high rate of mortality. Surgical intervention was invasive and almost uniformly fatal. The modern bronchoscope has undergone several modifications, including the addition of the rod-lens telescope by Harold Hopkins and the cold illumination source by Karl Storz in the 1950s to allow for improved visualization. In addition, the introduction of optical grasping forceps has improved therapeutic application, particularly with regard to foreign-body retrieval. With new technology and better anesthetic techniques, the diagnosis and management of pediatric airway disorder has improved significantly.

INDICATIONS FOR AIRWAY ENDOSCOPY

The indications for diagnostic or therapeutic airway bronchoscopy in the pediatric population are numerous. In children, rigid bronchoscopy is useful in the diagnosis and treatment of a variety of airway disorders from the larynx to the proximal bronchi. For examination of the bronchial tree beyond the carina and mainstem bronchi, flexible bronchoscopy has become the preferred tool for evaluating respiratory disorders in children. Indications for flexible bronchoscopy include, but are not limited to, patients with stridor, unresolving and recurring pneumonitis, persistent atelectasis, cough, tracheoesophageal fistula, airway trauma and tumor, and suspicion of foreign body. In addition, flexible bronchoscopy is very useful for taking samples for bronchoalveolar lavage. **Box 1** summarizes the common indications for performing airway endoscopy in children.

In certain clinical scenarios, such as an obstructive foreign body or significant airway hemorrhage, the rigid bronchoscope has a distinct advantage of allowing for ongoing ventilation throughout. This feature provides airway security and the time necessary to effectively diagnose and treat the airway problem. Furthermore, rigid bronchoscopy can facilitate endotracheal intubation and the Hopkins telescope can function as a guiding obturator for endotracheal tube placement via the Seldinger technique.[1]

Additional therapeutic capabilities of the rigid bronchoscope include dilation of stenosis or scar, marsupialization or debulking of cysts or tumors (cold, cautery, laser, or other techniques), biopsy of lesions, brushing for cytology/broncheoalveolar lavage specimens, stent placement, and retrieval of foreign bodies (**Fig. 1**). Visualization during foreign-body retrieval is greatly facilitated by using optical grasping forceps with an appropriate Hopkins rod. **Fig. 2** shows a common setup from rigid bronchoscopy for foreign-body removal.

FLEXIBLE VERSUS RIGID BRONCHOSCOPY

The flexible bronchoscope has emerged as an invaluable diagnostic and therapeutic tool with several advantages over the rigid bronchoscope. The flexible bronchoscope

| **Box 1** |
| **Indications for airway endoscopy in children** |
| Stridor |
| Airway foreign body |
| Caustic injury |
| Recurrent croup |
| Pneumonia |
| Atelectasis |
| Tracheomalacia or bronchomalacia |
| Stenosis or scar |
| Trauma |
| Mucus plugging |
| Tumors or other airway/mediastinal lesions |
| Suspected congenital airway anomaly |
| Management of the difficult pediatric airway |
| Bronchoalveolar lavage |
| Hemoptysis or pulmonary hemorrhage |
| Chronic cough |
| Tracheostomy evaluation and management |

is less invasive, can be used under local anesthesia or sedation, and provides improved visualization of the distal airways including a dynamic assessment during the respiratory cycle. Alternatively, the rigid bronchoscope allows for simultaneous ventilation and clear inspection of the larynx and subglottis, and is often required for more complicated instrumentation of airway lesions or foreign bodies. The therapeutic applications of the flexible bronchoscope are steadily increasing, however, with the development of airway balloons, electromagnetic technology and cryotechnology, laser technology, endobronchial ultrasound-guided biopsy, and others.[2,3] That being said, immediate availability of the rigid bronchoscope and an airway surgeon is critical when flexible techniques prove unsuccessful. **Table 1** provides a simple comparison of flexible and rigid endoscopy techniques for various assessments in children.

Both rigid and flexible bronchoscopy play an important role in the management of the difficult pediatric airway.[4–6] Independent of the type of endoscopy used, manipulating the pediatric airway requires meticulous preparation and clear, consistent communication between the proceduralist and the anesthesiologist.

EQUIPMENT FOR AIRWAY ENDOSCOPY
Rigid Bronchoscope

The rigid bronchoscope is available in several brands and sizes; however, its general morphology is similar. It consists of a solid metal tube, open on each end and containing multiple ports. The pediatric rigid bronchoscope is shorter and has a smaller diameter than those used in adults. The length is between 16 and 30 cm with an internal diameter from 3.2 to 7 mm. The thickness of the tube itself measures 2 to 3 mm, which must be added to obtain the external diameter. The Storz pediatric bronchoscope

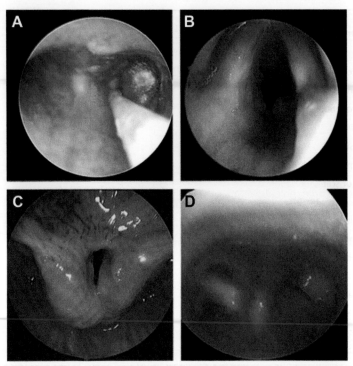

Fig. 1. (*A*) Rigid bronchoscopy for management of a right mainstem foreign body, highlighting the advantage of simultaneous ventilation, visualization, and intervention. (*B*) Subglottic cysts in an infant with stridor. (*C*) Supraglottic scarring secondary to intubation trauma during infancy as visualized with a Hopkins telescope during rigid bronchoscopy. (*D*) Bilateral mainstem foreign bodies diagnosed and extracted via rigid bronchoscopy.

sizes range from a 2.5 to 6. Size 2.5 has an external diameter of 4.2 mm whereas size 6 is 8.2 mm. It is important to choose the appropriately sized rigid bronchoscope for a patient based on age and size to minimize airway trauma (**Table 2**).

Hopkins Telescope

The Hopkins telescope may be used by itself to visualize the airway. This method is preferred by many surgeons for diagnostic bronchoscopy when the airway is easily exposed and the risk of oxygen desaturation during the procedure is low. When the Hopkins telescope is used in conjunction with the bronchoscope, it attaches via an adapter to the working port. Using this gasket creates a seal to allow continuous ventilation during the procedure. The Hopkins rod comes in multiple lengths and diameters. It is important to select a Hopkins telescope of the appropriate length and diameter to properly fit each bronchoscope. The appropriately sized telescope should sit just proximal to the beveled tip of the bronchoscope. In addition, there should be adequate space around the rod to allow for ventilation and passage of flexible suction or other necessary devices. It is noteworthy that narrower-diameter telescopes have an increased propensity to bend and fracture the optics. The telescope itself attaches to a light cord and source. In addition, the proximal telescope may be attached to a camera to allow for better visualization. **Fig. 2** shows Hopkins telescopes.

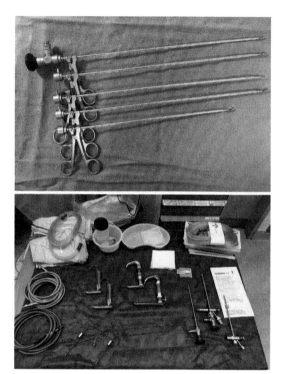

Fig. 2. Rigid bronchoscopy set up for foreign-body extraction in a child. Upper photo shows a Hopkins telescope with various sizes of laryngeal forceps to aid in foreign-body removal. Lower photo shows a variety of suspension laryngoscopes and rigid bronchoscopes of various diameters.

Flexible Fiberoptic Laryngoscope and Bronchoscope

Flexible instrumentation has revolutionized the way one diagnoses and treats problems in the pediatric airway. The caliber and length vary, with sizes ranging from 2.2 to 6.3 mm. The flexible laryngoscope is primarily a diagnostic tool and has no working channel. The fiberoptic bronchoscope is a flexible instrument, which is capable of transmitting an image from the distal tip to the proximal end. The combined characteristics of flexibility and image transmission permit clinicians to use this device as an aid to tracheal intubation and as a therapeutic instrument. Fiberoptic-guided tracheal intubation remains the gold standard for intubating the trachea in children with a difficult

Table 1		
Comparison of flexible and rigid endoscopy in children		
Assessment/Intervention	**Flexible**	**Rigid**
Laryngeal/glottic function	++	+
Bronchoalveolar lavage/bronchial biopsies	++	+
Subglottic disorder	+	++
Therapeutic interventions	+	++

++, clear benefit; +, some benefit.
Adapted from Nicolai T. Pediatric bronchoscopy. Pediatr Pulmonol. 2001;31:150-164; with permission.

Table 2
Tracheal tube and rigid bronchoscope sizes for children

Age	Airway Diameter (mm)	Tracheal Tube Size (mm)		Bronchoscope Size		
		ID	ED	Size	ID (mm)	ED (mm)
Premature	4.0	2.5–3.0	3.5–4.0	2.5	3.2	4.0
Term newborn	4.5	3.0–3.5	4.0–4.9	3.0	4.2	5.0
6 mo	5.0	3.5–4.0	4.9–5.4	3.0	4.2	5.0
1 y	5.5	4.0–4.5	5.4–6.2	3.5	4.9	5.7
2 y	6.0	4.5–5.0	6.2–6.9	3.5	4.9	5.7
3 y	7.0	5.0–5.5	6.9–7.4	4.0	5.9	6.7
5 y	8.0	5.5–6.0	7.4–7.9	5.0	7.0	7.8

Note that for premature infants and children with other medical comorbidities known to potentially affect the structure or caliber of the airway, bronchoscope sizes should be adjusted appropriately.
Abbreviations: ED, external diameter; ID, internal diameter.

airway.[7] In addition, fiberoptic laryngoscopy can be performed in the office-based setting using these thin flexible scopes while the patient is awake for diagnostic purposes (eg, locating foreign bodies, masses, or cysts in the pharynx and/or airway).

PHARMACOLOGIC/ANESTHETIC MANAGEMENT DURING AIRWAY ENDOSCOPY
Flexible Bronchoscopy

A combination of topical anesthetic and mild sedation with agents that maintain spontaneous ventilation (dexmedetomidine, fentanyl, ketamine, and/or midazolam) is often sufficient for flexible bronchoscopy. Lidocaine 2% to 4% spray will anesthetize the airway while midazolam and/or fentanyl is administered intravenously for sedation. Clinicians should be cognizant about the maximum safe doses of lidocaine in small children because they can easily be achieved given the smaller patient population. A maximal dose of 6 mg/kg is often used to limit the potential for local anesthetic toxicity. It should be recognized that premature neonates and small infants may have less protein binding of local anesthetic, thus predisposing them to local anesthetic toxicity. In these patients, a dose of 3 mg/kg may suffice to provide anesthesia. However, clinicians should use their judgment when deciding on an adequate dose of local anesthetic required for an infant, and they should base their decision on the factors governing absorption of local anesthetic and the patient's age, weight, and comorbidities.

In patients who are unable to tolerate a procedure under sedation, general anesthesia with an advanced airway may be necessary. During flexible bronchoscopy, a patient's airway can be managed with a supraglottic airway (SGA), an endotracheal tube (ETT), or an endoscopy mask. Compared with bag-mask ventilation, the former 2 methods provide more direct access to the trachea, and insertion of an ETT provides a more secure airway and a reliable means to provide positive-pressure ventilation in the lungs during therapeutic interventions. Nevertheless, in smaller children, bronchoscopy through an ETT is restricted to smaller-diameter bronchoscopes. Compared with ETTs, SGAs provide visualization of the supraglottic and laryngeal structures and allow the use of larger-diameter flexible bronchoscopes.[8] Regardless of which airway management option is chosen, it is important to have a deep plane of anesthesia to minimize reflex activation of the airway (coughing, bearing down, laryngospasm, bronchospasm), which can also lead to foreign-body dislodgment. Topical local anesthesia and/or titrated doses of opioids may help accomplish this.

Rigid Bronchoscopy

In children, sevoflurane is the pharmacologic agent of choice for mask induction and maintenance of anesthesia when rigid bronchoscopy is performed. Sevoflurane is preferred because it poses a lower risk for cardiac arrhythmias than halothane, which is still used in many developing countries. Spontaneous ventilation is often maintained during rigid bronchoscopy. Intravenous anesthetics such as propofol, dexmedetomidine, ketamine, and/or remifentanil are becoming increasingly popular for anesthesia maintenance because they provide a more reliable level of anesthesia that does not depend on native patient ventilation. When volatile agents are used alone, air leakage around the rigid bronchoscope may lead to a lighter plane of anesthesia, which may interfere with surgical manipulations while also contaminating the room with inhalation anesthesia. Intravenous anesthetic maintenance is less likely to affect anesthetic depth in comparison with volatile agents. It has been shown that fewer adverse events occur when intravenous anesthesia with propofol and remifentanil is used in combination with sevoflurane when compared with the use of sevoflurane alone during rigid bronchoscopy with spontaneous ventilation.[9] Nevertheless, both inhaled and intravenous methods are effective means by which anesthesia can be delivered to children undergoing rigid bronchoscopy.

FOREIGN-BODY REMOVAL BY RIGID BRONCHOSCOPY
Controlled Versus Spontaneous Ventilation for Rigid Bronchoscopy

The ventilating rigid bronchoscope can be used with spontaneous or controlled breathing. With either technique, once anesthesia is induced, local anesthesia (typically 1%–4% lidocaine) can be sprayed onto the epiglottis, larynx, and between the vocal cords to prevent laryngospasm and coughing, and decrease the general anesthetic requirements.

Mode of Ventilation: Spontaneous Versus Controlled Ventilation

Maintaining adequate ventilation and control of the airway is essential during interventional rigid bronchoscopy. Choosing whether to maintain spontaneous ventilation or initiate controlled ventilation is a difficult decision for clinicians because both methods have advantages and disadvantages. For example, in comparison with positive-pressure ventilation, spontaneous ventilation is less likely to advance the foreign body more distally, which would make removal of the object more challenging. Under controlled ventilation, the patient experiences brief periods of apnea as the operator maneuvers through the airway; by contrast, ventilation is uninterrupted if the patient is allowed to breathe spontaneously. Spontaneous ventilation, however, is associated with higher risk of patient movement and reflex activation of the airway (coughing, bearing down, laryngospasm, and bronchospasm), which can make foreign-body removal more arduous and can potentially lead to additional complications. These complications can often be managed by increasing the depth of anesthesia with an intravenous agent, such as propofol, or neuromuscular blocking drugs. Topicalization of the tracheobronchial tree with local anesthesia will also help to blunt airway reflexes. In addition to its lower risk of patient movement and airway reactivity, controlled ventilation may decrease atelectasis and hypercarbia, thus improving oxygenation. Advantages and limitations of controlled and spontaneous ventilation techniques during foreign-body extraction are compared in **Table 3**.

Table 3
Comparison of controlled and spontaneous ventilation for rigid bronchoscopy during foreign-body removal

Spontaneous Ventilation		Controlled Ventilation	
Advantages	**Disadvantages**	**Advantages**	**Disadvantages**
• Decreased risk of foreign-body dislodgment/movement • Better V/Q matching, less air trapping • Easier to oxygenate/ventilate through bronchoscope during manipulation of foreign body	• Increased risk of reflex activation of the airway (eg, laryngospasm, coughing), hypercarbia, and patient movement	• Decreases atelectasis • Associated with shorter operative times • Less potential for hypercarbia • Rapid airway control in case of full stomach	• Prolonged emergence from anesthesia • Increased risk of foreign-body dislodgment with positive-pressure ventilation • Intermittent apnea during removal

Abbreviation: V/Q, ventilation/perfusion.

To date, research to determine whether controlled or spontaneous ventilation is more beneficial during foreign-body removal has been inconclusive. Although controlled ventilation is associated with shorter operative times, the incidence of oxygen desaturation is not significantly different between the two, according to a meta-analysis.[10] In most cases, preserving spontaneous ventilation initially may be the safest method to prevent dislodgment of the foreign body. The anesthesiologist can later convert to controlled ventilation if necessary. More research is necessary to determine which modality of ventilation is better for both the bronchoscopist and the patient.

Technique for Foreign-Body Removal

Removal of a foreign body from a pediatric airway requires precision and dexterity. Bronchoscopy enables the clinician to locate and visualize the object, but various types of forceps and other instruments are used for retrieval. Forceps selection is typically based on the shape and nature of the foreign body. Once the bronchoscopist has established a secure grasp on the object, the forceps, object, and bronchoscope are removed simultaneously.

Inadvertent release of the foreign body during removal is a potentially life-threatening complication, as objects in the proximal airway may cause complete airway obstruction. In this situation, it may be best to push the object more distally into the bronchus from which it originated to preserve at least partial ventilation. The bronchoscopist can then regrasp the foreign body and make a second attempt at removal.

To facilitate removal and reduce the risk of accidently dropping the object, the clinician should relax the vocal cords with topical lidocaine or a muscle relaxant. The bronchoscope, forceps, and foreign body can then pass through the trachea and larynx more easily. After the object is successfully removed, a second bronchoscopy is usually performed to check for remnants of the foreign body that may have separated during the extraction and to assess for any airway damage.

Oxygenation During Airway Endoscopy

In small children, particularly infants, the tidal volume is fixed, functional residual capacity is less than closing capacity, and oxygen consumption is higher than in older children and adults. All of these physiologic variables lead to rapid oxygen desaturation with apnea under anesthesia. Indeed, the most common complication during pediatric difficult airway management is hypoxemia.[6]

Apneic oxygenation in the form of a nasal cannula may be useful during rigid bronchoscopy to minimize the risk of oxygen desaturation. In certain clinical scenarios including diagnostic bronchoscopy and foreign-body extraction, airway evaluation and intervention are carried out with the Hopkins telescope and forceps alone. In this scenario, oxygen delivery via nasal cannula or an endotracheal tube resting above the larynx can support the patient and add valuable time for diagnostic or therapeutic intervention.

Low-Flow Versus High-Flow Nasal Cannula Use During Airway Endoscopy

Both low-flow and high-flow techniques have been shown to be effective in pediatric patients. The nasal cannula is a well-tolerated, noninvasive device that delivers supplemental oxygen via soft prongs placed in the nares. The standard or low-flow nasal cannula (LFNC) can provide oxygen at rates of 1 to 10 L/min; however, prolonged use or flow rates greater than 2 L/min can cause nasal irritation or injury. An LFNC also cannot provide a sufficiently high oxygen concentration for severely hypoxemic patients. Although there are limited data on the use of the LFNC in pediatrics, it is effective in maintaining systemic oxygen saturation and prolonging apnea times.[11]

The high-flow nasal cannula (HFNC) delivers oxygen at rates that exceed a person's flow demands (up to 60 L/min), and delivers positive pressure for lung recruitment and the establishment of alveolar ventilation. The HFNC has only recently been applied to airway management in anesthesia.[12,13] It has been shown that in spontaneously breathing children with abnormal airways, maintenance of oxygenation during anesthesia for tubeless airway procedures is possible using an HFNC.[14]

Studies in adults have reported that an HFNC can prolong apneic times in the range of 50% to greater than 100%.[15,16] Apnea times are prolonged even at lower concentrations of oxygen, which may be necessary in tubeless airway surgery for safety concerns. Studies use the term transnasal humidified rapid-insufflation ventilatory exchange (THRIVE) to imply that an HFNC may not only provide oxygenation but may also help eliminate carbon dioxide.[15,16] The data are mixed regarding its ability to achieve ventilation in children.[12,17]

Once research can more clearly define optimal flow rates,[17] the use of apneic oxygenation could be expanded significantly to safely perform a wide range of surgeries. Apneic oxygenation is a technique that provides oxygenation, and possibly ventilation, without instrumentation of the airway, and has been shown to be effective in managing difficult airways and for use in airway surgery. **Fig. 3** shows a patient receiving HFNC during airway endoscopy.

Complications of Airway Endoscopy

The risk of complications varies based on underlying airway pathology, type and difficulty of therapeutic intervention, experience of the surgeon, and the patient's medical comorbidities. The most common complications are related to oxygenation and ventilation. Patients may become hypoxic or hypercapnic, which can lead to bradycardia and, possibly, cardiac arrest. Barotrauma can occur (eg, pneumothorax, pneumomediastinum) from inadequate egress of air from insufflation of oxygen during bronchoscopy. Fortunately, the mortality rate for both flexible and rigid endoscopy in the pediatric population remains fairly low.

Introduction of the laryngoscope, Hopkins telescope, or bronchoscope can damage the teeth, gingiva, or surrounding soft tissue. It is important to be aware of the

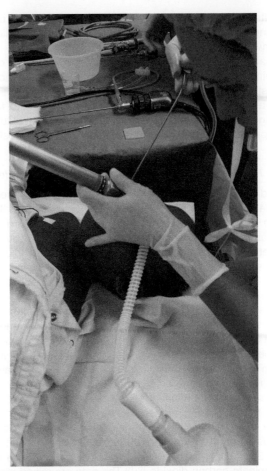

Fig. 3. Use of THRIVE high-flow nasal oxygenation in a 2-year-old child for direct laryngoscopy/rigid bronchoscopy. A high-flow nasal cannula may be useful to minimize the risk of oxygen desaturation during therapeutic rigid bronchoscopy.

bronchoscope position with regard to the lips and teeth to avoid pinching the lip with the scope or hitting the teeth. In addition, downward force should not be placed onto the maxillary teeth with the bronchoscope. A tooth guard or saline-soaked gauze and adequate hand positioning can help to minimize this risk. If dentition is damaged, a dental consult should be acquired. When placing tooth guards or gauze in the airway, it is critical to communicate this to the anesthesiologists and endoscopy nurses and to ensure their removal before emergence, otherwise airway aspiration and airway obstruction can occur.

When passing the bronchoscope, gentle maneuvering around the soft tissue of the posterior pharyngeal wall and epiglottis is important to avoid laceration and/or laryngeal fracture. In addition, there may be damage to the arytenoids or vocal folds when traversing this area. Ensuring that the bronchoscope passes through abducted vocal cords, posteriorly and at a 90° angle, can help to minimize laryngeal trauma. Significant trauma from the bronchoscope itself or from the therapeutic intervention could potentially induce a pneumothorax. If a pneumothorax is suspected, all operating room staff should be made aware of the situation, a chest film obtained immediately, and the appropriate surgical team consulted for chest tube placement.

DISCUSSION OF THE CASE PRESENTATION

The ear/nose/throat (ENT) surgeon decides to proceed with rigid bronchoscopy under general anesthesia for the removal of the foreign body from the right mainstem bronchus. Anesthesia is induced with sevoflurane via a mask, and titrated doses of fentanyl are administered before the rigid bronchoscope is placed. The rigid bronchoscope is then inserted into the trachea, and anesthesia is maintained with intravenous propofol. Oxygenation is possible through the rigid bronchoscope while spontaneous ventilation is maintained. When the ENT surgeon attempts to extract the foreign body with laryngeal forceps, the child coughs vigorously, leading to foreign-body dislodgment and a sudden inability to ventilate the lungs. Oxygen saturation decreases precipitously to 60%. Succinylcholine is administered intravenously, and an airway examination reveals that the foreign body is lodged in the lower trachea above the carina. The ENT surgeon then uses the rigid bronchoscope to advance the foreign body into the right mainstem bronchus to permit one-lung oxygenation and ventilation. After oxygen saturations improve, the foreign body is successfully extracted under controlled ventilation through the rigid bronchoscope. The postoperative course is uncomplicated and the child is discharged home.

SUMMARY

Rigid bronchoscopy and flexible bronchoscopy have an established role in various clinical scenarios for children, and are increasingly being used for both diagnostic and therapeutic purposes. Communication between the anesthesiologist and the airway endoscopist to ensure that adequate oxygenation and ventilation is maintained via the shared airway is of utmost importance, and will likely improve outcomes in this challenging population.

REFERENCES

1. Michaelson PG, Mair EA. Seldinger-assisted videotelescopic intubation (SAVI): a common sense approach to the difficult pediatric airway. Otolaryngol Head Neck Surg 2005;132:677–80.
2. Miller RJ, Casal RF, Lazarus DR, et al. Flexible bronchoscopy. Clin Chest Med 2018;39:1–16.
3. Zhang L, Yin Y, Jing Zhang J, et al. Removal of foreign bodies in children's airways using flexible bronchoscopic CO_2 cryotherapy. Pediatr Pulmonol 2016;51: 943–9.
4. Cohen S, Pine H, Drake A. Use of rigid and flexible bronchoscopy among pediatric otolaryngologists. Arch Otolaryngol Head Neck Surg 2001;127:505–9.
5. Weiss M, Engelhardt T. Proposal for the management of the unexpected difficult pediatric airway. Paediatr Anaesth 2010;20:454–64.
6. Fiadjoe JE, Nishisaki A, Jagannathan N, et al. Airway management complications in children with difficult tracheal intubation from the Pediatric Difficult Intubation (PeDI) registry: a prospective cohort analysis. Lancet Respir Med 2016;4:37–48.
7. Jagannathan N, Sohn L, Fiadjoe JE. Paediatric difficult airway management: what every anaesthetist should know! Br J Anaesth 2016;117(Suppl. 1):i3–5.

8. Baker PA, Brunette KE, Byrnes CA, et al. A prospective randomized trial comparing supraglottic airways for flexible bronchoscopy in children. Paediatr Anaesth 2010;20:831–8.

9. Chai J, Wu XY, Han N, et al. A retrospective study of anesthesia during rigid bronchoscopy for airway foreign body removal in children: propofol and sevoflurane with spontaneous ventilation. Paediatr Anaesth 2014;24:1031–6.

10. Liu Y, Chen L, Li S. Controlled ventilation or spontaneous respiration in anesthesia for tracheobronchial foreign body removal: a meta-analysis. Paediatr Anaesth 2014;24:1023–30.

11. Olayan L, Alatassi A, Patel J, et al. Apnoeic oxygenation by nasal cannula during airway management in children undergoing general anaesthesia: a pilot randomised controlled trial. Perioper Med (Lond) 2018;7. https://doi.org/10.1186/s13741-018-0083-x.

12. Riva T, Pedersen TH, Seiler S, et al. Transnasal humidified rapid insufflation ventilatory exchange for oxygenation of children during apnoea: a prospective randomised controlled trial. Br J Anaesth 2018;120:592–9.

13. Humphreys S, Lee-Archer P, Reyne G, et al. Transnasal humidified rapid-insufflation ventilatory exchange (THRIVE) in children: a randomized controlled trial. Br J Anaesth 2017;118(2):232–8.

14. Humphreys S, Rosen D, Housden T, et al. Nasal high-flow oxygen delivery in children with abnormal airways. Paediatr Anaesth 2017;27:616–20.

15. Patel A, Nouraei SA. Transnasal Humidified Rapid-Insufflation Ventilatory Exchange (THRIVE): a physiological method of increasing apnoea time in patients with difficult airways. Anaesthesia 2015;70:323–9.

16. Mir F, Patel A, Iqbal R, et al. A randomised controlled trial comparing transnasal humidified rapid insufflation ventilatory exchange (THRIVE) pre-oxygenation with facemask pre-oxygenation in patients undergoing rapid sequence induction of anaesthesia. Anaesthesia 2017;72:439–43.

17. Jagannathan N, Burjek N. Transnasal humidified rapid-insufflation ventilatory exchange (THRIVE) in children: a step forward in apnoeic oxygenation, paradigm-shift in ventilation, or both? Br J Anaesth 2017;118(2):150–2.

Partnership with Interventional Pulmonologist

An Anesthesiologist's Perspective

Wendy M. Suhre, MD[a],*, John D. Lang Jr, MD[a],
David K. Madtes, MD[b], Basem B. Abdelmalak, MD[c,d]

KEYWORDS

- Nonoperating room anesthesia • Anesthesia techniques
- Interventional pulmonology • Bronchoscopy

KEY POINTS

- Interventional procedures requiring nonoperating room anesthesia, including bronchoscopy, have increased significantly over the last decade.
- Patients presenting for interventional bronchoscopic procedures often have many comorbidities that increase the risks associated with anesthesia, and therefore require a thorough assessment prior to the procedure.
- Anesthetic type, medications, and airway choices depend on patient factors and type of procedure.
- Complications of interventional bronchoscopic procedures include airway fire, barotrauma, intrapulmonary hemorrhage, and damage to airway structures.

INTRODUCTION

There has been an enormous growth in interventional procedures conducted over the last decade and interventional pulmonology is no exception.[1] While many of the recent advances allow patients to forgo more aggressive surgeries, the procedures themselves are generally technically ambitious and are occurring in patients of greater age and medical complexity. This, coupled with improved anesthetic techniques and improved technology, has led up to 30% of anesthetics being delivered outside

[a] Department of Anesthesiology and Pain Medicine, University of Washington School of Medicine, 1959 NE Pacific St, BB-1469, Box 356540, Seattle, WA 98195-6540, USA; [b] Medicine Department, Division of Pulmonary and Critical Care Medicine, University of Washington School of Medicine, 1100 Fairview Ave. North, Campus Box 35080 (D3-190), Seattle, WA 98109-1024, USA; [c] Department of General Anesthesiology, Anesthesiology Institute, Cleveland Clinic, Cleveland, OH 44195, USA; [d] Department of Outcomes Research, Anesthesiology Institute, Cleveland Clinic, 9500 Euclid Avenue, Cleveland, OH 44195, USA
* Corresponding author.
E-mail address: suhre@uw.edu

Otolaryngol Clin N Am 52 (2019) 1049–1063
https://doi.org/10.1016/j.otc.2019.08.006
0030-6665/19/© 2019 Elsevier Inc. All rights reserved.

of the classic operating room (OR) setting, a term commonly referred to by anesthesiologists as NORA (nonoperating room anesthesia). In this setting, the anesthesiologist faces unique challenges that include geographic dislocation from more familiar areas such as the OR and postanesthesia care unit (PACU), suboptimal space, substandard work ergonomics, and finally procedural and personnel unfamiliarity.[2] In this article, the goal will be to lay out the expanding partnership between the interventional pulmonologist and anesthesiologist, from the anesthesiologist perspective. In doing so, the authors hope that this will enhance familiarity and ultimately facilitate a more cohesive team approach in the provision of quality care to a complex patient population.

THE EVOLVING NONOPERATING ROOM ANESTHESIA SETTING

The authors' local experience has been consistent with others in that OR volume remains relatively flat (1%–2% per year), but NORA volumes are growing rapidly. With this growth has come the need for enhanced familiarity and day-to-day joint collaboration not only in the care of patients, but also in the planning of current and future work space, patient scheduling and work flow, allocation of anesthesiology resources, adherence to safety and efficiency metrics, and expectation of preprocedural patient work-up and postprocedural care. Progress has been made with the commitment of many individuals from differing backgrounds working together as a team. Thus, many health care facilities have put together a governing group to oversee and ensure that care provided in NORA locations is standardized and of the highest quality and safety.[2,3]

Because of the consistent need for anesthesiologist services, many centers are attempting to retrofit suites to allow more space to fit anesthesia service needs, such as increasing room capacity, more strategic placement of critical gases, increasing the number of electrical outlets, allowing for the permanent presence of anesthesia delivery systems, and ensuring appropriate anesthetic scavenging systems.[4] To this point, the additional ripple requires the expanded footprint of other critical personnel such as anesthesia technicians. They work alongside anesthesiologists to guarantee the case-to-case availability of standardized anesthesia carts with specialty equipment including devices for addressing difficult airways and cardiopulmonary resuscitation. This necessitates an expanded footprint for the anesthesia technician to ensure timely supply replacement and to assist the anesthesiologist with other needs that may arise. To complement timely administration of an anesthetic whether that be sedation and/or general anesthesia, close proximity of an automated medication dispensing system is also necessary.

Postinterventional patient care and personnel workflow should also be emphasized. NORA growth has placed significant demand on fixed capacity areas such as the postanesthesia care units (PACUs) and intensive care units (ICUs), normally considered high-volume areas for traditional surgical patients. Growth estimates should be carefully considered to ensure the appropriate patient:bed ratios so as to not compromise safety and efficient work flow. To address this challenge, many NORA sites have established their own recovery space following procedures requiring anesthesia (phase 1 recovery).

In the past, patient scheduling of NORA cases had been a rare random occurrence because of the paucity of volume and unpredictability of the need for an anesthesiologist. This, along with an improper scheduling system, inevitably led to a patient/provider being disadvantaged because of lack of anesthesiology availability. As procedures have advanced and volumes grown, the need for anesthesia services has grown to the point that more rational approaches to scheduling had to be adapted to enhance predictable access, maximize efficiency, and increase financial productivity. As opposed to irregular and random schedules, predictable blocks of time (ie, 10 hours) are allocated on given days to allow for enhanced productivity, efficiency, and satisfaction. Procedures are scheduled sequentially to reduce underutilized time and ensuring anesthesia coverage. Advantages include predictable allocated time, reduced patient/provider waiting time, enhanced financial benefit, and improved patient/provider satisfaction. Utilization of this block is followed at frequent intervals and is expanded or reduced based on the utilization rate (ie, a target of 70% to 80% is desirable). Moreover, by conforming to block scheduling, there is significant aligning of processes regarding anesthesiology oversight and responsibility over patient safety, quality, and operational efficiency in the OR and NORA. This has recently allowed anesthesiologists to implement and enforce their protocols that ensure a methodical and thorough safety checklist that is conducted on every patient. Quality metrics for each subspecialty NORA area are tracked. Efficiency metrics such as on-time first case starts, procedure turnover times, procedure delays, and cancellations are also tracked in conjunction with the ORs. Historically, NORA sites have performed poorly compared with the main OR suite; however, since there has been an emphasis on alignment and transparency in metrics' sharing, the gaps have narrowed. Because of variability in patient acuity, uniqueness of many of the cases being performed, and work flow challenges, it is probably an unrealistic expectation that NORA efficiency will reach that of the OR.

Ideally, all NORA cases should be scheduled using the same software as surgical procedures. This results in much fewer scheduling problems that may delay access and create staff/provider conflict. All scheduled NORA procedures should be displayed alongside the standard surgical schedule on all official scheduling systems. This ensures that NORA procedures are equal emphasis to the operating room. In fact, with the current trend, NORA case volumes will soon consistently account for close to half of the daily case volume requiring anesthesia.

RISKS OF SEDATION AND ANESTHESIA IN NONOPERATING ROOM ANESTHESIA

Anesthesiologists have proven crucial in improving patient safety. In fact, the National Patient Safety Foundation based its model on the Anesthesia Patient Safety Foundation. The American Society of Anesthesiology closed claims database (cases litigated and claims paid) has been used as a source of reporting sedation and anesthetic risks.[5] In 2009, Metzner and colleagues reported that the incidence of claims arising from anesthesia care conducted in NORA locations had significantly higher proportion of deaths compared with the OR. Most of these were respiratory-related. The most common anesthetic technique being used was sedation, albeit at varying depths, so commonly referred to as monitored anesthesia care (MAC). In addition, respiratory depression secondary to oversedation and polypharmacy (propofol combined with sedatives/analgesics) accounted for over one third of the claims. The same trend has been reported by other investigators also.[6] Complications when deep sedation is provided by nonanesthesiologists have been reported to be even higher.[7] More recently, Chang and colleagues[8] examined the National Anesthesia Clinical Outcomes Registry database and compared anesthetic complications in OR procedures versus NORA procedures, which did not include bronchoscopic procedures (n = 12,252,846 cases). This analysis found that major complications (defined as need for escalation in care, need for respirator, need for resuscitation, and serious hemodynamic instability) were higher in OR versus NORA cases. Moreover, overall mortality was significantly higher in OR versus NORA cases. An important point to note, however, is that when gastroenterology patients were taken out of the analysis, NORA case mortality was significantly greater. Interestingly, wrong patient/side procedures were also higher in NORA cases, reinforcing the point that adherence to universal protocols to ensure patient safety is still in need of improvement. Certainly, future investigations should continue to prospectively assess causality and solutions to specific complications encountered in NORA cases. It is incumbent on anesthesiologists to partner with hospital leadership and interventionalists in determining the optimal care delivery models.

PREPROCEDURAL WORK-UP

Patients presenting for interventional pulmonology procedures are generally classified as American Society of Anesthesiology physical status (ASA PS) 3 or greater (in fact a great percentage of them are justifiably ASA PS 4). Preoperative assessment should be performed as is done for any other patient with significant comorbidities. This includes a thorough airway examination and an inquiry of existing symptoms of airway compromise. History and physical examination should focus on evaluation of acute and chronic conditions. Focused questions to the patient regarding shortness of breath, exercise tolerance, cough and recent infections, smoking history, diagnosis of chronic obstructive pulmonary disease, and use of bronchodilators or steroids should be posed. Inquiring about previous chemotherapy is important, particularly the use of bleomycin and its associated risks for pulmonary fibrosis and acute oxygen toxicity, as well as doxorubicin and its potential for causing cardiomyopathy. Patients may exhibit signs for chronic hypoxemia such as cyanosis and/or clubbing. Functional capacity, respiratory rate and pattern, and pulmonary auscultation can help gauge the degree of respiratory compromise. Review of available pulmonary function testing, arterial blood gas, and selected radiology imaging can be helpful. In addition, the pulmonologist's evaluation of the lesion/tumor and its location, as well as the degree of impact on ventilation should be reviewed and shared with the anesthesiologist. The likelihood of a difficult airway in these patients is not increased compared with any average surgical patients; however, lower airway related difficulties may be encountered including airway bleeding, obstruction, or loss of airway integrity. Many of these patients have a history of cardiac disease, necessitating the need to ensure that the patient has no active/unstable cardiac conditions. Certain techniques such as rigid bronchoscopy require neck hyperextension, so patients presenting for this procedure should be assessed for risk factors for cervical spine subluxation.

ANESTHESIOLOGISTS' INTERPRETATION OF INTERVENTIONAL (DIAGNOSTIC AND THERAPEUTIC) BRONCHOSCOPIC PROCEDURES

Bronchoscopic procedures are often done on individuals with multiple comorbidities and can present a challenge to the anesthesiologist and the pulmonologist.[9] It is important to understand the procedure to be performed, and the underlying pathology, in order to deliver a safe and successful anesthetic. A summary of the anesthetic need for such procedures is shown in **Box 1**.

ANESTHETIC PHARMACOLOGY
Sedatives/Anxiolysis

Sedatives and anxiolytics such as midazolam should be used carefully, especially in patients with advanced degrees of respiratory compromise because of the risk for respiratory depression. Of note, oversedation with benzodiazepines also can lead to

Box 1	
Summary of the anesthetic need for various procedures	
Procedure	**Anesthetic**
Flexible diagnostic bronchoscopy	Moderate to deep sedation, general anesthesia
Rigid bronchoscopy	General anesthesia
Endobronchial ultrasonography	General anesthesia; can be done with moderate-to-deep sedation; however, general anesthesia is advantageous
Airway laser procedures	General anesthesia, lowest possible Fio_2 to avoid airway fire
Electromagnetic navigation bronchoscopy	General anesthesia; can be done with moderate to deep sedation; however, general anesthesia is advantageous

disinhibition, complicating a bronchoscopic procedure that could otherwise be performed in a lightly sedated and cooperative patient. Supplemental oxygen should be considered before administering any sedatives, and anxiolytics should be used in only extremely anxious patients. Oral clonidine (150 mcg or up to 3 mcg/kg) may also be employed because of its sedative effect and ability to blunt the hemodynamic response to bronchoscopy and/or laryngoscopy. However, clonidine use for this indication has not gained much popularity.

Corticosteroids

A 24-hour course of dexamethasone or other corticosteroid has been proposed to reduce laryngeal edema and decrease postextubation stridor or obstruction in the ICU.[10,11] Although there is no documented evidence that the use of corticosteroids has any benefit in relationship to airway swelling in bronchoscopic procedures, many practitioners administer dexamethasone (5–10 mg) intravenously to prevent airway swelling based on clinical merits in cases of longer duration or when extensive inflammation of vocal cords or airway mucosa is expected or visualized. These relatively small doses administered over a short duration have proven to be safe.

Antiemetic Agents

Aspiration during and after bronchoscopic interventions is a real possibility. Because many of the patients undergoing such procedures have limited pulmonary reserve, aggressive postprocedural nausea and vomiting prophylaxis is probably warranted. This is complex subject matter and varies depending on patient risks factors, history of adverse effects, costs, and drug availability. One hard and fast rule is that treatment should be administered with an antiemetic from a pharmacologic class that is different from the prophylactic drug initially given, or if no prophylaxis was given, the recommonded treatment is a low-dose 5-HT3 antagonist.[12,11]

Antacids and Prokinetics

Gastric acidity reduction may decrease the risk for pneumonitis and/or pneumonia in patients who aspirate, although no evidence supports its routine use. Protein pump inhibitors are the most potent class, but take up to a day to work. Thus, they have no real role as a true preoperative medication. In contrast, histamine-2 (H2) antagonists may produce a clinically significant increase in gastric pH and reduction in gastric volume 30 to 60 minutes after an intravenous dose or 2 to 3 hours after an oral dose.

Metoclopramide is often used as a prokinetic in patients with gastroparesis. Less effective in increasing gastric pH than H2 blockers, metoclopramide also has potential adverse effects and drug and disease interactions, making it a less attractive option. In patients with high aspiration risk presenting without sufficient time for other medications to take effect, a nonparticulate antacid such as 0.3 M sodium citrate can be administered with a resultant immediate increase in gastric pH.

Bronchodilators

Patients with asthma or chronic obstructive pulmonary disease (COPD) with a reversible component generally receive a preprocedure short-acting bronchodilator, but this may not produce any benefit in COPD. Atropine possesses protective bronchodilatory properties when given before bronchoscopic procedures; however, it can produce secondary tachycardia that may be detrimental in patients with coronary artery disease.

Local Anesthesia in Preparations for Bronchoscopic Procedures

Bronchoscopy in a patient not receiving general anesthesia requires adequate suppression of airway reflexes to facilitate the procedure. The degree and location of necessary reflex suppression depend on the planned airway management and route of bronchoscopy. Perineural injections, topicalization with local anesthetics, or a combination of these techniques may be used. In any case, lidocaine is the preferred local anesthetic because of its rapid onset, short duration of action, and relative safety.

Nasal Anesthesia

Adequate nasal anesthesia usually can be achieved using a combination of a topical decongestant, such as oxymetazoline or phenylephrine, followed by application of viscous lidocaine jelly. This regimen usually provides adequate sensory blockade and lubrication to allow passage of a nasal trumpet, bronchoscope, or endotracheal tube (ETT). Alternatively, the pterygopalatine ganglion (providing sensory input to the anterior third of the nasal septum and posterior nasal cavity) can be blocked by soaking a cotton ball or cotton-tipped applicator in 2% to 4% lidocaine with epinephrine (1:200,000), 4% cocaine, or phenylephrine (1:20,000), passing it slowly to the posterior wall of the nasopharynx, and leaving it in place for 5 to 10 minutes.

Anesthesia of the Posterior Oropharynx and Upper Airway

To tolerate awake/sedated techniques for either nasotracheal or orotracheal bronchoscopy or intubation, sequential blockade of the superior laryngeal nerve and recurrent laryngeal nerve is required, via either perineural injections or via mucosal saturation. Direct regional blockade of the superior laryngeal nerve is performed bilaterally at the level of the thyrohyoid membrane, just inferior to the greater cornu of the hyoid bone. A small-bore needle is directed anteroinferomedially until the greater cornu is contacted; the needle is then withdrawn slightly, and after negative aspiration is confirmed, 2 mL of 2% lidocaine is injected. The block is repeated in the same fashion on the contralateral side.

To suppress coughing, anesthesia to the recurrent laryngeal nerve is required when the bronchoscope is passed through the vocal cords and into the trachea and can be readily achieved by translaryngeal block. A 20- or 22-gauge needle on a syringe under constant negative pressure is advanced through the cricothyroid membrane until air is aspirated, and then 4 mL of 2% to 4% lidocaine with epinephrine are injected. Patients invariably cough with the delivery of the local anesthetic solution, which helps disperse the local anesthetic but increases the risk for puncturing the back wall of the trachea with the needle.

Although direct regional blockade is most reliable, adequate anesthesia usually can be achieved with topical local anesthetic application and mucosal saturation. 5 mL of 4% lidocaine or another local anesthetic can be aerosolized via a standard nebulizer attached to a face mask or mouthpiece and are well tolerated in nearly all patients. With enough time, aerosolized local anesthetic usually provides adequate initial anesthesia of the oropharynx and upper airway. Although most have abandoned its use, benzocaine spray can be used, but excessive administration is a well-known cause of methemoglobinemia.

Finally, the channel of a flexible bronchoscope can be used to sequentially spray 1 to 2 mL of 2% to 4% lidocaine on the epiglottis, vocal cords, and carina. Systemic lidocaine levels are generally negligible even when administered to mucosa using a combination of methods, but should not exceed 8 mg/kg body weight to reduce the risk of local anesthetic toxicity.

ANESTHETIC APPROACHES FOR INTERVENTIONAL PULMONARY PROCEDURES

When considering the anesthetic approach for bronchoscopic procedures, the anesthesiologist must consider the type of anesthetic, airway device needed, and ventilation to be used depending upon the particular procedure to be performed and patient comorbidities.[9,15] If premedication is used, careful titration should be employed, as these patients can be sensitive to any respiratory depression. The addition of an antisialogogue such as glycopyrolate may be considered.

Choice of Anesthetic

Monitored anesthesia care

MAC does not describe the continuum of depth of sedation. Rather it describes a specific anesthesia service in which an anesthesiologist has been requested to participate in the care of a patient undergoing a diagnostic or therapeutic procedure. MAC may include varying levels of sedation, analgesia, and anxiolysis as necessary. During MAC, the anesthesiologist is prepared to convert to general anesthesia when necessary. MAC can be used for uncomplicated diagnostic or simple therapeutic flexible bronchoscopic procedures in patients who do not have significant pulmonary compromise and are likely to tolerate the procedure without ventilation support.

Sedation

Flexible bronchoscopy performed in an otherwise healthy patient will generally not require anything more than moderate sedation along with airway reflex suppression via any of the previously described techniques. A combination of intravenous fentanyl titrated over the duration of the procedure in 12.5- to 50-mcg aliquots (2–2.5 µg/kg) with midazolam 0.5 to 2 mg (total) usually provides adequate sedation, anxiolysis, and some cough suppression. Anesthesiologists will more commonly utilize propofol, and if administered will be either by intermittent boluses (10–20 mg) or as a low-dose infusion (10–50 mcg/kg/min).[16–18] Compared with the combination of midazolam and fentanyl, propofol allows for more rapid recovery and easier titration in bronchoscopic cases lasting for longer intervals (20–30 min). Remifentanil can also be employed as monotherapy for moderate sedation or as an infusion following a 0.5 to 2 mg titration of midazolam. The initial infusion rate should be 0.1 mcg/kg/min for patients 65 years or younger started 5 minutes prior to bronchoscopy, with the infusion then weaned to approximately 0.05 mcg/kg/min as tolerated during the procedure.[19] This will generally provide satisfactory sedation and cough suppression for bronchoscopy and has even been used for more stimulating procedures, such as tracheoplasty using combined laser and balloon dilation. Remifentanil offers an advantage as a sole agent over other opioids, because patients predictably awaken within 4 to 5 minutes of discontinuation of its infusion, regardless of infusion duration. As with most narcotics, respiratory depression, chest wall rigidity, and laryngospasm are potential serious complications of remifentanil, but they are reversible with naloxone.

The α-2 agonist dexmedetomidine has been utilized as a sedative agent for bronchoscopic procedures. This agent requires a loading infusion, typically 0.5 to 1 mcg/kg over 10 to 20 minutes, before the initiation of a maintenance infusion of 0.2 to 1.0 mcg/kg/h[19,20] Given the relatively short duration and fast turnover of most procedures performed in an interventional suite, this relatively long loading time may not be cost-effective or efficient in high-volume centers. With that said, dexmedetomidine is appealing, because it assists in maintaining upper airway patency and respiratory center output in addition to providing analgesia and acting as an antidelirium agent. Dexmedetomidine can cause bradycardia and hypotension, so one should be wary of these effects.

Lastly, inhalation of helium (70% or more) along with oxygen is occasionally needed for patients with upper airway obstruction. Helium's reduced density compared with that of oxygen allows for enhanced laminar flow and increased velocity, thus can assist in reducing respiratory effort and improving oxygen delivery (**Fig. 1**).[21]

General anesthesia

Induction General anesthesia may be necessary for longer cases, procedures where immobility is necessary, or when significant stimulation is anticipated.

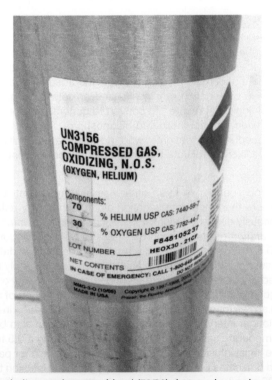

Fig. 1. A tank of a helium and oxygen blend (70/30) that can be used as an adjunct to assist in patients with airway obstruction during bronchoscopic procedures.

Like the OR, propofol at 1 to 2 mg/kg is one of the most commonly used primary induction medications in a bronchoscopy suite. Other agents may also be utilized. For instance, etomidate administered at 0.2 to 0.3 mg/kg is an alternative induction agent for patients with impaired left ventricular function; however, there have been concerns regarding suprarenal suppression in patients suffering from severe sepsis or septic shock. Ketamine is another agent that may be utilized because of its unique characteristics. As an indirect sympathomimetic, it may bronchodilate and assist in preserving respiratory drive and cardiac function at an induction dose of 1 to 2 mg/kg. However, its undesirable side effects, including hallucination and emergence delirium, can be ameliorated with the use of a benzodiazepine (eg, midazolam 1–2 mg). Complete opioid-based or benzodiazepine-based induction regimens are rarely appropriate for bronchoscopic procedures, because the doses required to achieve adequate anesthetic depth do not allow emergence in a timely manner. Inhaled sevoflurane may be used to gently induce general anesthesia in cases of large anterior mediastinal masses with the objective of maintaining spontaneous ventilation.

Maintenance of general anesthesia Total intravenous anesthesia (TIVA) or inhalational anesthetic can be employed for maintenance of general anesthesia, although TIVA is probably preferred for bronchoscopic procedures. Most notably, repeated insertion and removal of the bronchoscope with the resulting circuit leak cause interrupted delivery of volatile agents. TIVA ensures uninterrupted, thus reliable, delivery of anesthesia independent of ventilation and avoids exposing procedural room personnel to inhalational agent. Additional advantages of a propofol-based TIVA include less postoperative nausea and vomiting, decreased cough on induction and emergence, and less depression of bronchial mucous transport velocity.[22] Inhalational anesthetics may at least theoretically predispose patients to increased bleeding at the site of needle puncture during biopsies, likely because of local vasodilation in the bronchial mucosa from the volatile agent. Propofol may be used as the lone agent for maintenance of anesthesia for flexible bronchoscopy at a dose of 75 to 250 mcg/kg/min. Recovery of consciousness is quick and generally predictable after short cases typical of bronchoscopic procedures. If a target-controlled infusion is employed (not available in the United States), appropriate induction and maintenance plasma concentration targets for propofol are 7 mcg/mL and less than 5 to 6 mcg/mL, respectively. This is done in conjunction with remifentanil infusion or intermittent fentanyl boluses.[23] To help monitor the depth of anesthesia and decrease the risk of awareness, electro-encephalographic monitors such as the Bispectral Index Monitor (BIS Monitor, Medtronic, Dublin, Ireland) may be considered. In some instances, an inhalational anesthetic may be the preferred agent used. This may be the case when the maintenance of spontaneous respirations is required as in the resection of anterior mediastinal masses, tracheoesophageal fistulae repair, or for cases requiring transpulmonary biopsies. The use of general anesthesia also allows for the use of muscle relaxants regardless of the airway used (endotracheal tube or supraglottic airway).

Muscle relaxation Most procedures performed in the bronchoscopy suite can be done without pharmacologic muscle relaxation if optimal conditions can be achieved by other means. Advantages of forgoing neuromuscular blockade include no chance of residual paralysis or recurarization of patients with baseline or anticipated limited pulmonary reserve after the procedure. However, many interventionalists and anesthesiologists prefer muscle relaxation for these procedures (regardless of the airway choice), especially in those with a high risk for airway injury or hemorrhage or the potential for spontaneous respiratory effort against an obstructed or occluded airway, which can lead to negative-pressure pulmonary edema. Special attention to neuromuscular monitoring and reversal of neuromuscular agents is critical, especially in shorter procedures. The desirable benefits of muscle relaxation in routine bronchoscopic procedures include the ease and atraumatic insertion of the airway (endotracheal tube [ETT]/supraglottic airway or rigid bronchoscope), minimal trauma (from the procedural flexible and/or rigid bronchoscope) to the vocal cords and the airway in general, patient stability for accurate biopsying, and higher yield with the least number of needle insertions. Muscle relaxation as a part of a balanced anesthetic technique can help minimize the required infused dose of propofol, and eliminates the need for the concomitant use of a potent narcotic such as remifentanil or vasopressor agents to maintain hemodynamic stability.

Choice of Airway

Choosing the type of airway depends upon the procedure to be performed, location of the lesion, and needs of the pulmonary team. Options include a natural airway, supraglottic airway, endotracheal tube, rigid bronchoscope, and an existing airway such as a cuffed tracheostomy tube.

Natural airway
A natural airway is a good choice for MAC/sedation cases, especially those performed in a bronchoscopy suite that does not have an anesthesia machine. When using a natural airway, adequate topical anesthesia must be used to allow patients to tolerate the procedure without the need for deep sedation while maintaining spontaneous ventilation. Humidified high-flow oxygen through a nasal cannula (HFNC) in combination with remifentanil and propofol infusions has been shown to be effective for bronchoscopy and endobronchial ultrasound (EBUS), although further studies are needed to determine correct flow rates and level of sedation.[24]

Endotracheal tube
Advantages to using an ETT include the delivery of continuous ventilation during bronchoscopy, protection from aspiration risk, and avoidance of vocal cord trauma as the bronchoscope is passed in and out of the airway (**Fig. 2**). Intubation with a large-diameter ETT (8.0–9.0 mm ID) allows for adequate ventilation of the patient around the large diameter flexible scope while avoiding high airway pressures. Sometimes, the proximal end of the ETT may be cut to shorten the overall length of the ETT and facilitate bronchoscope maneuverability; however, for some cases, the full length of the ETT is needed to advance into a main bronchus for single-lung ventilation if bleeding in the airway from a highly vascular tumor occurs.[25] A fiberoptic swivel adaptor is commonly used to allow continuous ventilation and avoid disconnection of the circuit during the procedure; however, high flows are generally needed to compensate for the unavoidable air leak in the circuit.

Supraglottic airway
A superglottic airway (SGA) can be helpful in EBUS mediastinal staging procedures, as it allows for biopsy of station 2 nodes that are located high in the tracheobronchial tree. SGAs are also a good choice for patients with subglottic tracheal lesions, because the SGA does not enter the glottis and is therefore out of the surgical field (**Figs. 3** and **4**). The SGA acts as a conduit for the FOB and provides a means of ventilation (**Fig. 5**). Moreover, SGAs seem to be reliable options for metallic stent removals when the stent is located high in the trachea and intubation with an ETT would be risky. The SGA is not a definitive airway, may not seat properly in select patients, shares some of the ETT

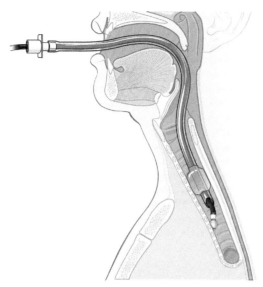

Fig. 2. A secured ETT can serve as a protected conduit to the distal trachea and below. (Reprinted with permission, Cleveland Clinic Center for Medical Art & Photography © 2011-2019. All Rights Reserved.)

complications such as airway trauma (eg, laryngospasm, sore throat), and does not protect against aspiration (**Fig. 6**).

Rigid bronchoscope

This is a helpful airway in certain situations such as inserting and/or removing silicone stents, as well as part of the management of patients with anterior mediastinal masses and/or central airway obstruction. During rigid bronchoscopy, ventilation is achieved with attachment of the anesthetic circuit to the side port on the bronchoscope or via jet ventilation, with the jet ventilator also attached to the bronchoscope through the side port with an adaptor. Leaks are common, but may be overcome with high flows or packing the oral pharynx with saline-soaked gauze when positive pressure ventilation is utilized. This packing should be periodically removed to allow egress of air and avoid pulmonary barotrauma.

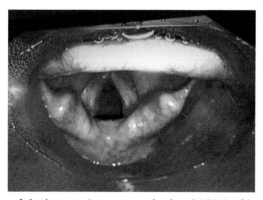

Fig. 3. Visualization of the larynx using as properly placed SGA, in this case, an I-gel.

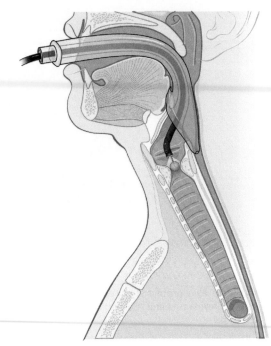

Fig. 4. An SGA airway can be successfully utilized in patients with tracheal obstruction. (Reprinted with permission, Cleveland Clinic Center for Medical Art & Photography © 2011-2019. All Rights Reserved.)

Fluid administration

Fluid administration should be kept to a minimum to avoid pulmonary congestion and precipitate cardiogenic or noncardiogenic pulmonary edema in these patients with little lung reserve and possibly concomitant cardiac disease.

Complications of bronchoscopic procedures

Potential complications of these procedures include hypercarbia, hypoxemia, and cough, as well as devastating situations including loss of airway, bleeding, airway fire, pneumothorax, and injury to the larynx or airway structures.[26] Use of jet ventilation can be complicated by pulmonary barotrauma. With the use of argon and Nd:YAG lasers, cerebral and cardiac air emboli have been reported.

Airway fire

Airway fires are of among the most devastating complications of interventional bronchoscopic procedures. If a fire occurs, several steps should be taken:

1. Turn off the O_2
2. Remove ETT
3. Flush the area with water/saline, including the airway
4. Reintubate immediately and resume ventilation with 100% O_2
5. Assess the damage to the airways with a bronchoscope and remove residual debris and consider cold water lavage
6. Administer antibiotics and consider intravenous steroids
7. Continue supportive therapy

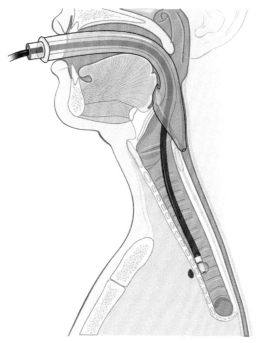

Fig. 5. An SGA, like an ETT, can be used as a conduit to the distal tracheal and below. (Reprinted with permission, Cleveland Clinic Center for Medical Art & Photography © 2011-2019. All Rights Reserved.)

Intrapulmonary hemorrhage

Bronchoscopy-induced bleeding requiring intervention can occur in approximately 2% to 5% of patients.[26] There is an increased risk of bleeding in patients undergoing a transbronchial biopsy and on antiplatelet medications (eg, Plavix) and have an uncorrected coagulopathy or are thrombocytopenic. Many techniques have been described to control the bleeding, including ice cold saline lavage; endobronchial irrigation with epinephrine/norepinephrine (low dose in small aliquots), both administered through the bronchoscope; tamponade with a balloon or the bronchoscope itself; and

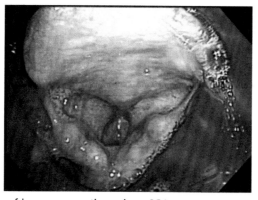

Fig. 6. Visualization of laryngospasm through an SGA.

laser or electrocautery if available. Epinephrine may precipitate coronary spasm and induce arrhythmias and should not be used in patients with coronary artery disease, arrhythmias, or carcinoid tumors. Several small studies have described the use of tranexamic acid applied directly to the biopsy site, which was effective for hemostasis.[27–29] For continued bleeding despite these interventions, a double-lumen tube may be placed; the tracheal cuff will act as a barrier to the blood, and the bronchial cuff will protect the contralateral lung.

SUMMARY

Tremendous growth and change are ongoing in NORA sites, and interventional pulmonology is no exception. In order to be successful, it is crucial to work as a cohesive team to ensure patient safety. The anesthesiologist serves as a great teammate for the interventional pulmonologist and offers expertise that is complementary to the success of cutting-edge pulmonary interventional techniques.

REFERENCES

1. Arias S, Lee HJ. The future of interventional pulmonology. Semin Respir Crit Care Med 2014;35(6):763–8.
2. Caplan JP, Querques J, Epstein LA, et al. Consultation, communication, and conflict management by out-of-operating room anesthesiologists: strangers in a strange land. Anesthesiol Clin 2009;27(1):111–20.
3. Eichhorn V, Henzler D, Murphy MF. Standardizing care and monitoring for anesthesia or procedural sedation delivered outside the operating room. Curr Opin Anaesthesiol 2010;23(4):494–9.
4. Pino RM. The nature of anesthesia and procedural sedation outside of the operating room. Curr Opin Anaesthesiol 2007;20(4):347–51.
5. Metzner J, Posner KL, Domino KB. The risk and safety of anesthesia at remote locations: the US closed claims analysis. Curr Opin Anaesthesiol 2009;22(4):502–8.
6. Cravero JP. Risk and safety of pediatric sedation/anesthesia for procedures outside the operating room. Curr Opin Anaesthesiol 2009;22(4):509–13.
7. Vargo JJ, Holub JL, Faigel DO, et al. Risk factors for cardiopulmonary events during propofol-mediated upper endoscopy and colonoscopy. Aliment Pharmacol Ther 2006;24(6):955–63.
8. Chang B, Kaye AD, Diaz JH, et al. Interventional procedures outside of the operating room: results from the National Anesthesia Outcomes Registry. J Pat Safe 2018;14(1):9–16.
9. Abdelmalak BB, Gildea TR, Doyle DJ. Anesthesia for bronchoscopy. Curr Pharm Des 2012;18(38):6314–24.
10. Francois B, Bellissant E, Gissot V, et al. 12-h pretreatment with methylprednisolone versus placebo for prevention of postextubation laryngeal oedema: a randomised double-blind trial. Lancet 2007;369(9567):1083–9.
11. Jaber S, Jung B, Chanques G, et al. Effects of steroids on reintubation and postextubation stridor in adults: meta-analysis of randomised controlled trials. Crit Care 2009;13(2):R49.
12. Golembiewski J, Tokumaru S. Pharmacological prophylaxis and management of adult postoperative/postdischarge nausea and vomiting. J Perianesth Nurs 2006; 21(6):385–97.

13. Kim EJ, Ko JS, Kim CS, et al. Combination of antiemetics for the prevention of postoperative nausea and vomiting in high-risk patients. J Korean Med Sci 2007;22(5):878–82.

14. Skolnik A, Gan TJ. Update on the management of postoperative nausea and vomiting. Curr Opin Anaesthesiol 2014;27(6):605–9.

15. Pawlowski J. Anesthetic considerations for interventional pulmonary procedures. Curr Opin Anaesthesiol 2013;26(1):6–12.

16. Clark G, Licker M, Younossian AB, et al. Titrated sedation with propofol or midazolam for flexible bronchoscopy: a randomised trial. Eur Respir J 2009;34(6): 1277–83.

17. Lo YL, Lin TY, Fang YF, et al. Feasibility of bispectral index-guided propofol infusion for flexible bronchoscopy sedation: a randomized controlled trial. PLoS One 2011;6(11):e27769.

18. Stolz D, Kurer G, Meyer A, et al. Propofol versus combined sedation in flexible bronchoscopy: a randomised non-inferiority trial. Eur Respir J 2009;34(5): 1024–30.

19. Ryu JH, Lee SW, Lee JH, et al. Randomized double-blind study of remifentanil and dexmedetomidine for flexible bronchoscopy. Br J Anaesth 2012;108(3): 503–11.

20. Bergese SD, Patrick Bender S, McSweeney TD, et al. A comparative study of dexmedetomidine with midazolam and midazolam alone for sedation during elective awake fiberoptic intubation. J Clin Anesth 2010;22(1):35–40.

21. Conacher ID. Anaesthesia and tracheobronchial stenting for central airway obstruction in adults. Br J Anaesth 2003;90(3):367–74.

22. Hohlrieder M, Tiefenthaler W, Klaus H, et al. Effect of total intravenous anaesthesia and balanced anaesthesia on the frequency of coughing during emergence from the anaesthesia. Br J Anaesth 2007;99(4):587–91.

23. Prakash N, McLeod T, Gao Smith F. The effects of remifentanil on haemodynamic stability during rigid bronchoscopy. Anaesthesia 2001;56(6):576–80.

24. Service JA, Bain JS, Gardner CP, et al. Prospective experience of high flow oxygen during bronchoscopy in 182 patients: a feasibility study. J Bronchology Interv Pulmonol 2018;26(1):66–70.

25. Abdelmalak B, Sethi S, Gildea TR. Anesthesia and upper and lower airway management for advanced diagnostic and therapeutic bronchoscopy. Adv Anesth 2014;32(1):71–87.

26. Lee P, Mehta AC, Mathur PN. Management of complications from diagnostic and interventional bronchoscopy. Respirology 2009;14(7):940–53.

27. Zamani A. Bronchoscopic intratumoral injection of tranexamic acid: a new technique for control of biopsy-induced bleeding. Blood Coagul Fibrinolysis 2011; 22(5):440–2.

28. Zamani A. Bronchoscopic intratumoral injection of tranexamic acid to prevent excessive bleeding during multiple forceps biopsies of lesions with a high risk of bleeding: a prospective case series. BMC Cancer 2014;14:143.

29. Marquez-Martin E, Vergara DG, Martin-Juan J, et al. Endobronchial administration of tranexamic Acid for controlling pulmonary bleeding: a pilot study. J Bronchology Interv Pulmonol 2010;17(2):122–5.

Regional Anesthesia and Acute Pain Management

Garrett Burnett, MD*, Samuel DeMaria Jr, MD, Adam I. Levine, MD

KEYWORDS

- Regional anesthesia • Acute pain management • Nerve block
- Multimodal analgesia

KEY POINTS

- Multimodal analgesia techniques use regional anesthesia blocks with a variety of medications that provide analgesia through different biochemical pathways.
- Regional anesthesia may provide intraoperative and postoperative analgesia, which decreases opioid requirements in the perioperative period.
- Team work throughout the perioperative period between the otolaryngologist and anesthesiologist is vital for providing quality acute pain management.

INTRODUCTION

Postoperative pain is a common preoperative concern of patients undergoing surgery, and approximately 75% of patients report moderate to extreme pain in the immediate postoperative period. In addition, adverse effects from postoperative pain medications, such as opioids, are common (**Table 1**).[1,2] Collaboration between otolaryngologists and the anesthesiologists is vital in improving acute pain management in ear, nose, and throat surgery by using regional anesthesia and multimodal analgesia techniques.

CONTENT
Background

Acute pain can be defined as "the physiologic response and experience to noxious stimuli that can become pathologic, is normally sudden in onset, time limited, and motivates behaviors to avoid actual or potential tissue injuries."[3] Historically, acute pain management relied on opioid medications given intermittently or via a patient-controlled analgesia device throughout the perioperative period. Because of the current opioid crisis within the United States, a greater interest in opioid-sparing

Department of Anesthesiology, Perioperative and Pain Medicine, Icahn School of Medicine at Mount Sinai, 1468 Madison Avenue, 8th Floor, New York, NY 10029, USA
* Corresponding author.
E-mail address: garrett.burnett@mountsinai.org

Otolaryngol Clin N Am 52 (2019) 1065–1081
https://doi.org/10.1016/j.otc.2019.08.013
0030-6665/19/© 2019 Elsevier Inc. All rights reserved.

Table 1 Adverse effects of opioids	
Nausea/Vomiting	Ileus
Pruritus	Urinary retention
Altered mental status	Confusion
Respiratory depression	Sedation
Immunomodulation	Androgen deficiency
Hyperalgesia	Sleep disturbances

Data from Benyamin R, Trescot AM, Datta S, et al. Opioid complications and side effects. Pain Physician. 2008;11(2 Suppl):S105-20 and Swegle JM, Logemann C. Management of common opioid-induced adverse effects. Am Fam Physician. 2006;74(8):1347-1354.

multimodal acute pain management has continued to develop within all fields of surgery, including otolaryngology.[4,5]

Acute Pain Management

Multimodal analgesia is the foundation for modern perioperative acute pain management. Multimodal analgesia involves the use of multiple medications and techniques to synergistically improve pain control while decreasing side effects associated with opioid pain medications.[6] Although the transition from acute pain to chronic pain does not regularly occur following a procedure, surgery may be the inciting trigger for chronic opioid use or abuse[7] (see **Table 1**).

Surgical stimulus causes the release of numerous inflammatory mediators, such as substance P, prostaglandins, histamine, bradykinin, and excitatory neurotransmitters. Multimodal analgesia is used to attack the multiple biochemical pathways that result in the release of these inflammatory mediators.

Preventive analgesia is the use of medications for pain to prevent peripheral and central sensitization to pain before the beginning of surgery. Preventive analgesia has replaced the prior term of preemptive analgesia because preventive analgesics may be given to the patient at any point in the perioperative period, including preoperatively. Preventive analgesia and multimodal analgesia work synergistically to improve postoperative pain and decrease analgesic consumption.[8]

Multimodal analgesia regimens may use any number of combinations of medications for treatment of acute pain, including nonsteroidal antiinflammatory drugs (NSAIDs), acetaminophen, anticonvulsants, corticosteroids, N-methyl D-aspartate (NMDA) receptor antagonists, antidepressants, and local anesthetics. The American Society of Anesthesiologists practice guidelines on acute pain management recommend multimodal analgesia with regional blockade and around-the-clock dosing of NSAIDs or acetaminophen when appropriate.[9] A list of common components of multimodal analgesia regimens and their methods of action are listed in **Table 2**.[10]

Nonsteroidal antiinflammatory drugs

NSAIDs are medications that inhibit the cyclooxygenase (COX)-1 and COX-2 enzymes from producing prostaglandins, such as prostaglandin E_2, which leads to inflammation and pain sensitization.[11] Parenteral or enteral formulations are available and examples of common NSAIDs include ibuprofen, ketorolac, and naproxen. NSAIDs have been shown to significantly decrease perioperative opioid use within various fields of surgery,[12–14] including otolaryngology.[15,16]

Adverse effects from NSAIDs have been attributed to inhibition of the COX-1 enzyme and include risk of renal dysfunction, gastrointestinal hemorrhage, and

Table 2
Multimodal analgesic drugs

Class	Mechanism	Examples
Nonsteroidal antiinflammatory	Inhibition of COX-1 and COX-2 enzymes	Ibuprofen, ketorolac, naproxen, celecoxib
Acetaminophen, paracetamol	Inhibition of central prostaglandin synthesis	Acetaminophen, paracetamol
Local anesthetics	Sodium channel blockers, which prevent neuronal depolarization	Lidocaine, mepivacaine, cocaine, bupivacaine, ropivacaine
Anticonvulsant	Voltage-dependent calcium channel inhibitor	Gabapentin, pregabalin
Corticosteroids	Glucocorticoid agonist	Dexamethasone
NMDA receptor antagonist	NMDA receptor antagonist, opioid receptor agonist	Ketamine
Opioids	Blockade of mu-opioid receptors	Fentanyl, hydromorphone, morphine, oxycodone

Abbreviation: COX, cyclooxygenase.
Data from Young AC, Buvanendran A. Multimodal analgesia: pharmacologic interventions and prevention of persistent postoperative pain. In: Hadzic A, ed. *Hadzic's Textbook of Regional Anesthesia and Acute Pain Medicine.* 2nd ed. New York: McGraw Hill; 2017:1219-1225.

platelet dysfunction.[17] Although platelet dysfunction and bleeding are a risk of NSAID use, NSIADs such as ketorolac and ibuprofen have not been shown to significantly increase bleeding in endoscopic sinus surgery,[18] thyroid surgery,[19] or adenotonsillectomy surgery.[15,16,20]

Because of these adverse effects associated with COX-1 inhibition, the COX-2 selective inhibitor celecoxib has been used for multimodal analgesia in otolaryngology. Celecoxib has been shown to significantly decrease pain and improve patient satisfaction with outpatient otolaryngologic surgery[21] as well as decrease the total opioid requirements with head and neck cancer procedures, including free tissue transfer.[22]

Acetaminophen

Acetaminophen produces analgesia via inhibition of central prostaglandin synthesis but has no effect on peripheral prostaglandin synthesis. In addition to analgesic effects, acetaminophen is a weak antiinflammatory drug.[23] Acetaminophen may be given in both enteral and parenteral forms effectively and is often given every 6 hours in the postoperative period. Within otolaryngology, acetaminophen has been shown to decrease postoperative opioid requirements for tonsillectomy procedures in children.[24] In addition, a combination of NSAID and acetaminophen provides more effective perioperative analgesia than acetaminophen alone.[21,25]

The maximum dose of acetaminophen is 4000 mg/d,[26] but should be limited to 3000 mg/d in patients with poor liver function.[10] Acetaminophen is the most common source of acute liver failure, which may be caused by intentional or unintentional overdose.[27] It is important to monitor for all sources of acetaminophen because it is commonly included in over-the-counter headache and cold medications. Unlike NSAIDs, acetaminophen does not have an effect on renal function, gastric mucosa, or platelet function.

Local anesthetics

Local anesthetics may be used in otolaryngology through infiltration or discrete nerve blocks (discussed later). Local anesthetics may be safely used as a primary anesthetic technique in otolaryngology[28] as well as for intraoperative and postoperative analgesia.[29–31] Evidence for the use of local anesthetics and regional anesthesia suggests its use may decrease chronic pain as well as hyperalgesia and central sensitization.[32,33] Both short-acting (eg, lidocaine, mepivacaine) and long-acting (eg, bupivacaine, ropivacaine) local anesthetics may be used for otolaryngologic procedures.

Local anesthetics function via inhibition of voltage-gated sodium channels within nerve fibers. Inhibition of voltage-gated sodium channels prevents nerve depolarization and propagation of impulses of sensory and motor signals.[34] Properties of local anesthetics such as pKa, lipid solubility, and protein binding affect clinical properties such as speed of onset, potency, and duration of action, respectively.[35] Newer controlled-release local anesthetics, such as liposomal bupivacaine, have been approved for local wound infiltration and certain nerve blocks. Liposomal bupivacaine is associated with a prolonged duration of action compared with plain bupivacaine.[36] Liposomal bupivacaine has not been investigated within otolaryngology and many existing studies have compared liposomal bupivacaine with saline, which may not be a reliable indicator of its efficacy.

Adjuvants may be added to local anesthetics to achieve various clinical effects. Epinephrine is a common local anesthetic adjuvant that prolongs sensory and motor blockade through vasoconstriction and direct alpha-2 agonism. The use of local anesthetics with epinephrine for regional anesthesia has been shown to improve surgical visualization during functional endoscopic sinus surgery.[37] Dexamethasone is a synthetic corticosteroid that may be added to local anesthesia in order to provide improved quality of block and prolonged analgesia through its antiinflammatory effects.[38] Alpha-2 agonists such as clonidine and dexmedetomidine may produce prolonged sensory and motor blockade through multiple mechanisms, such as local vasoconstriction[39] and direct local anesthetic properties.[40] Other additives, such as opioids, which are typically added to local anesthetics for intrathecal and epidural nerve blocks, have failed to show significant improvement in peripheral nerve block duration or quality.

Although typical doses of local anesthetics used within otolaryngology are not high, it is important to understand and recognize potential complications of local anesthetic administration (**Box 1**). One instance of high-dose local anesthetics in otolaryngology is the use of large doses of topical and infiltrated local anesthetics for awake intubation techniques.[41] In addition, because of the proximity of important structures in the head and neck region, intravascular injection of small amounts of local anesthetics may cause a greater effect, causing complications such as total spinal anesthetic or local anesthesia systemic toxicity (LAST). Maximum doses of commonly used local anesthetics are listed in **Table 3**. Recognition of LAST is important because lipid emulsion therapy as well as supportive care are vital in preventing morbidity and mortality[42] (see **Box 1**, **Table 3**).

Anticonvulsants
Anticonvulsants such as gabapentin and pregabalin have been shown to be beneficial in multimodal analgesia. Both drugs inhibit voltage-dependent calcium channels, which leads to decreased release of substance P and calcitonin gene–related peptide. Studies have shown a decreased opioid consumption postoperatively, earlier cessation of opioids postoperatively, and prevention of chronic pain.[45,46] Studies within otolaryngology support the use of anticonvulsants in the treatment of acute pain.[47,48]

Side effects may limit the use of anticonvulsants in multimodal analgesia. The most common side effects of these drugs include dizziness, somnolence, blurred vision, ataxia, weight gain, and fatigue. Reducing the dose of gabapentin or pregabalin may decrease these side effects.[10]

Box 1
Adverse effects of local anesthetic administration

Local Anesthetic Systemic Toxicity:
- Neurologic effects: tinnitus, circumoral numbness, metallic taste, agitation, seizures
- Respiratory effects: respiratory arrest
- Cardiovascular effects: ventricular arrhythmias, asystole, myocardial depression

Allergic reaction
- Rare, more common in ester-type local anesthetics

Methemoglobinemia

Damage to surrounding structures
- Nerve injury
- Bleeding/hematoma
- Injury to airway

Failed block:
- Incorrect technique
- Inadequate dosage
- Anatomic variation
- Acidic tissue

Infection

Pain on injection

Retained block needle

Total spinal anesthesia

Respiratory distress caused by phrenic or recurrent laryngeal nerve block

Data from Refs.[42–44]

Corticosteroids

Corticosteroids (eg, dexamethasone, hydrocortisone) modulate the inflammatory response to surgical stimuli within a multimodal analgesia technique. Incorporating corticosteroids into a multimodal analgesia regimen decreases postoperative pain and opioid use.[49] Dexamethasone has been shown to reduce pain, postoperative nausea and vomiting, bleeding, and overall complications following tonsillectomy.[50,51]

Table 3
Maximum doses of local anesthetics

Medication	Maximum Dose (mg/kg)	Duration (h)
Lidocaine	4.5	0.75–1.5
	7 (with epinephrine)	
Mepivacaine	4.5	1–2
	7 (with epinephrine)	
Prilocaine	8	0.5–1
Bupivacaine	3	1.5–8
Ropivacaine	3	1.5–8
Chloroprocaine	12	0.5–1
Procaine	12	0.5–1
Cocaine	3	0.5–1
Tetracaine	3	1.5–6

One important aspect of corticosteroids in otolaryngology is the reduction of airway and tissue edema.

Complications of corticosteroids include hyperglycemia, poor wound healing, gastrointestinal complications, and potential suppression of the hypothalamic-pituitary-adrenal axis.[10]

N-methyl D-aspartate receptor antagonists

NMDA receptor antagonists (eg, ketamine) provide multiple benefits for acute pain management, including reduction of acute postoperative pain, analgesic consumption, and the development of chronic pain.[52,53] In addition to NMDA receptor antagonism, ketamine affects numerous receptors, including agonism of mu, delta, and kappa opioid receptors. Ketamine has been shown to decrease postoperative pain following tonsillectomy through the intravenous[54] and topical[55] routes.

Although ketamine provides numerous benefits, side effects are common at high doses. Side effects include hallucinations, nightmares, cognitive dysfunction, and increased salivation. These side effects may be prevented through the use of lower doses of ketamine (<1 mg/kg), antimuscarinic drugs (eg, glycopyrolate), and benzodiazepines.[10,56]

Opioids

Although the goal of a multimodal analgesic regimen is to decrease the amount of opioid pain medications required following surgery, opioids are often required for pain control in the acute perioperative period. Opioids should be available to patients in the postoperative period for acute pain, but should be used with caution and their use restricted in quantity and duration.

Opioids decrease pain through activation of mu receptors in the central nervous system. Opioids may be pure agonists, partial agonists, or mixed agonist-antagonists. Pure agonists, such as fentanyl and morphine, are the most effective for acute pain management. Mixed agonist-antagonists may be used for treatment of chronic pain or addiction.[57]

Opioids may be delivered via patient-controlled analgesia system, intravenous bolus, or enteral formulations. As previously discussed, opioids are associated with numerous side effects, which may limit use (see **Table 1**), as well as potential for dependence or addiction.

Regional Anesthesia Techniques

Regional anesthesia has been used for dental procedures for many years and its use has continued to develop within otolaryngology. Regional anesthesia may be used for a primary anesthetic, perioperative analgesia, or to facilitate awake intubations in patients with difficult airways.

Although regional anesthesia is often beneficial, it is important to consider contraindications, such as patient refusal, infection at injection site, disorder involving area, coagulopathy (especially when site is not compressible), and inability to identify landmarks (obesity, postradiation changes, postsurgical changes). Injection of local anesthetic may also interfere with computed tomography guidance used for sinus and transsphenoidal surgeries; therefore, it is important to register the patient with the guidance software before injection of local anesthetic.[37]

Trigeminal nerve blocks

Sensory innervation of the face is supplied via branches of the trigeminal nerve (or cranial nerve V). The trigeminal ganglion lies in the Meckel cave and divides into

3 nerves: the ophthalmic (V1) nerve, the maxillary (V2) nerve, and the mandibular (V3) nerve.[44] These 3 nerves provide sensory innervation to the face, as shown in **Fig. 1**.

Ophthalmic (V1) nerve: supraorbital block The ophthalmic nerve is a sensory nerve that branches to form the lacrimal, frontal, and nasociliary nerves that supply the forehead, eyebrows, upper eyelids, and anterior aspect of the nose. The frontal nerve, the largest branch of the ophthalmic nerve, may be blocked at the supraorbital notch. Indications for supraorbital nerve block include surgeries involving the area of distribution, including lacerations, craniotomies, or ventriculoperitoneal shunt placement. Complications include hematoma, intravascular injection, and eye globe damage.

The supraorbital block begins with palpation of the supraorbital foramen along the superior medial aspect of the orbit. A 25-gauge needle is inserted toward the supraorbital notch and following negative aspiration 0.5 to 1.0 mL of local anesthetic is injected (**Fig. 2**). All figures of blocks in this article are simulated using a high-fidelity simulator mannequin.

Maxillary (V2) nerve: infraorbital and sphenopalatine blocks The maxillary nerve is a purely sensory nerve innervating the skin of the upper lip, lower eyelid, medial cheek, and lateral edges of the nose. Portions of the maxillary nerve may be blocked via the infraorbital block, as the maxillary nerve exits the infraorbital foramen,[44] or by the sphenopalatine block, which blocks the sphenopalatine ganglion. The sphenopalatine ganglion receives sensory innervation from the maxillary nerve as well as additional innervation from the facial nerve (cranial nerve VII).[58]

Infraorbital block The infraorbital block is indicated for cleft lip repair, lower eyelid procedures, endoscopic sinus surgery,[30] rhinoplasty, and transsphenoidal procedures. Complications include hematoma, persistent paresthesia, and intravascular injection.

The infraorbital block may be performed via the intranasal or intraoral route. Both techniques begin with palpation of the infraorbital foramen on the inferior medial orbital rim. For the intranasal approach, a 25-gauge needle is inserted through the

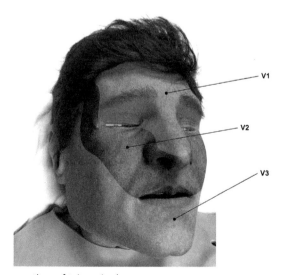

Fig. 1. Sensory innervation of trigeminal nerve.

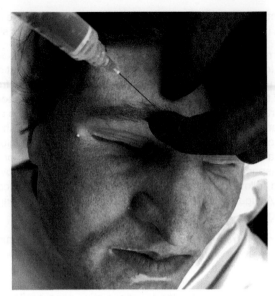

Fig. 2. Supraorbital block.

inside of the ipsilateral nare and directed toward the infraorbital foramen. After negative aspiration, 1 to 3 mL of local anesthetic is injected just before the foramen. For the intraoral approach, a 25-gauge needle is inserted into the buccal mucosa in front of the maxillary teeth and tunneled toward the infraorbital foramen. After negative aspiration, 1 to 3 mL of local anesthetic is injected just before the foramen[44] (**Fig. 3**).

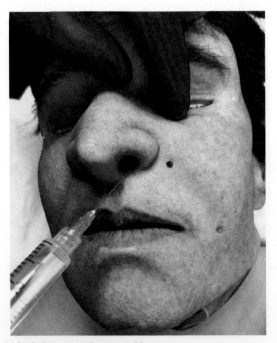

Fig. 3. Infraorbital block (intranasal approach).

Extreme care must be taken to avoid entering the infraorbital notch and traumatizing or injecting local anesthetic into the globe of the eye regardless of technique.[59]

Sphenopalatine block The sphenopalatine ganglion provides sensory innervation to the orbit, nose, buccal mucosa, palate, and paranasal sinuses.[37] It is used in functional endoscopic sinus surgery for analgesia,[31] reduction of postoperative nausea and vomiting,[60] and improved surgical visualization when combined with a vasoconstrictor. Complications of sphenopalatine ganglion block include intravascular injection, hematoma, diplopia, and infraorbital nerve injury.

The sphenopalatine block may be performed via the intraoral approach following induction of general anesthesia. The greater palatine foramen can be identified just medial to the gum line of the first or second molar on the posterior portion of the hard palate. Following negative aspiration with a 25-gauge needle, 1.5 to 2 mL of local anesthesia is injected through the foramen (**Fig. 4**). Injection into the hard palate should include a mild to moderate amount of resistance when injecting. If the injection is very easy, the injection may be into the soft palate. It is recommended that epinephrine 1:100,000 be added to reduce systemic absorption and improve surgical conditions via sphenopalatine artery vasocontriction.[37]

Mandibular (V3) nerve: inferior alveolar block The mandibular nerve is a sensory and motor nerve innervating the sensation of the front of the ear, temples, anterior two-thirds of the tongue, and mandible. The inferior alveolar block targets the mandibular nerve between the medial aspect of the ramus of the mandible and the lateral aspect of the sphenomandibular ligament. The lingual nerve is a branch of the mandibular nerve and is often blocked during the inferior alveolar block. Indications for inferior alveolar nerve block include surgery involving the mandible, mandibular teeth, floor of mouth, tongue, and lower lip or chin. Complications of inferior alveolar block include intravascular injection, hematoma, and block failure.

The inferior alveolar block is performed intraorally. With the patient's cheek retracted, the coronoid notch is identified or palpated and the pterygomandibular

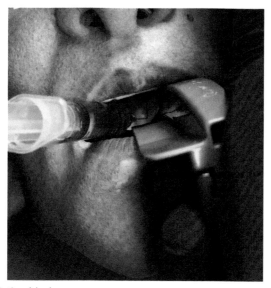

Fig. 4. Sphenopalatine block.

raphe is identified. A 25-gauge needle is inserted from the contralateral aspect of the mouth between the coronoid notch and the pterygomandibular raphe (**Fig. 5**). The needle is advanced until the mandible is contacted; the needle is then withdrawn 1 mm and 2 to 5 mL of local anesthetic is injected. In order to block the lingual nerve, an additional 2 to 4 mL of local anesthetic should be injected as the needle is withdrawn.[61]

Cervical plexus blocks The cervical plexus is composed of ventral rami from C1 to C4, which innervate the anterolateral neck, periauricular region, and skin overlying the medial aspect of the clavicle. The cervical plexus may be blocked using the superficial approach only and similar results are achieved with or without the deep block with significantly fewer side effects.

Indications for cervical plexus block include thyroidectomy, parathyroidectomy, tracheostomy, carotid endarterectomy, and superficial procedures of the neck. Significant complications of cervical plexus block, such as total spinal anesthesia and vertebral artery injection, are associated with deep cervical plexus blockade. Additional complications of cervical plexus block include intravascular injection, hematoma, and phrenic nerve paresis. Because of the risks associated with the deep cervical plexus block, the superficial cervical plexus block is preferred. Our institution has omitted the use of the deep cervical block.

The superficial cervical plexus block is performed by depositing 10 mL of local anesthetic along the length of the posterior portion of the sternocleidomastoid muscle (**Fig. 6**). The goal is to inject the local anesthetic superficial to the cervical fascia.[62] This block is commonly performed using a landmark-based technique but ultrasonography may be used to identify the superficial cervical plexus. The use of deep fanning of the needle at the midway point between the mastoid process and C6, as described in other sources, should be avoided because the brachial plexus can be injured.

Blocks for awake fiber-optic intubation Many patients presenting for head and neck surgery have disorders associated with difficult airways. These disorders may

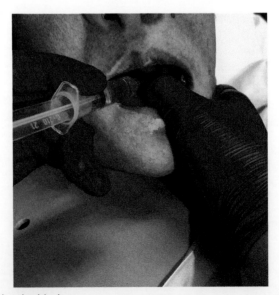

Fig. 5. Inferior alveolar block.

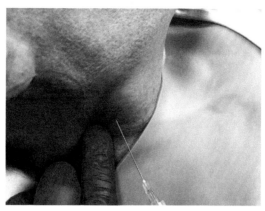

Fig. 6. Superficial cervical plexus block.

include head and neck cancer, large goiter, and prior head and neck surgery or radiation. The best practice for intubation of patients with difficult airways is an awake intubation typically using a flexible bronchoscope. Judicious topical local anesthetics to block the upper airway in combination with blocks of the vagus nerve (cranial nerve X) allow a smooth awake intubation with minimal patient discomfort.

Recurrent laryngeal nerve block The recurrent laryngeal nerve has motor and sensory function. The nerve supplies motor innervation to all muscles of the larynx except the cricothyroid and sensory innervation to the larynx below the vocal cords. There is significant risk for vocal cord paralysis and airway obstruction with a discrete block of the recurrent laryngeal nerve; therefore, a transtracheal approach is used to topicalize the region supplied by the recurrent laryngeal nerve. Complications of transtracheal recurrent laryngeal nerve block include intravascular injection, hematoma, and esophageal injury.

The recurrent laryngeal nerve block is performed by first identifying the cricothyroid membrane at the midline of the patient's anterior neck. Ultrasonography may be used to identify the cricothyroid membrane in patients with difficult anatomy (**Fig. 7**). The nondominant hand is used to stabilize the trachea and a small amount of local anesthesia is infiltrated overlying the cricothyroid membrane. A 20-gauge angiocatheter with its introducer needle in place is connected to a syringe containing 5 mL of lidocaine 4%. The needle is advanced through the skin and cricothyroid membrane until the airway is accessed (**Fig. 8**). Confirmation of placement can be done by aspirating

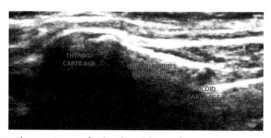

Fig. 7. Ultrasonography anatomy of cricothyroid membrane.

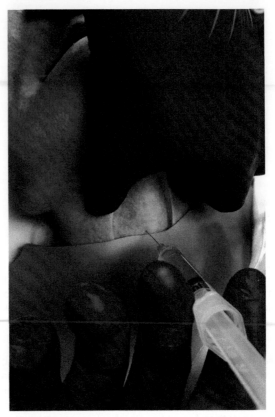

Fig. 8. Recurrent laryngeal nerve block.

bubbles of air. The angiocatheter is then threaded over the needle and the needle is removed. The local anesthetic is then injected through the catheter, which elicits coughing to distribute the local anesthesia. Alternatively, a 20-gauge needle may be used without the angiocatheter, but the angiocatheter allows decreased risk of injury during patient coughing and provides emergency access to the airway throughout the intubation.[63]

Superior laryngeal nerve block The superior laryngeal nerve block provides sensory innervation to the larynx above the vocal cords as well as motor innervation to the cricothyroid muscle. The nerve is located just inferior to the greater cornu of the hyoid bone where it splits into internal and external branches. Complications of the superior laryngeal nerve block include intravascular injection, hematoma, injury to surrounding structures, and block failure.

To perform the superior laryngeal nerve block, the hyoid bone must be identified using palpation or ultrasonography. If the hyoid bone is unable to be identified, the superior cornu of the thyroid cartilage may serve as a landmark. The hyoid bone is displaced using pressure from the contralateral side and a 25-gauge needle is advanced from the lateral aspect of the ipsilateral neck until contact is made with the hyoid bone. The needle is then moved inferiorly off the bone and 2 mL of local anesthetic is injected (**Fig. 9**). The block is the performed on the contralateral side to block the superior laryngeal nerve bilaterally.

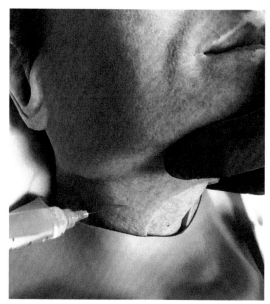

Fig. 9. Superior laryngeal nerve block.

SUMMARY

Multimodal analgesia with regional anesthesia provides improved pain control throughout the perioperative period for patients undergoing head and neck surgeries. Acute pain management with multimodal techniques is vital in the current era of opioid crisis. Teamwork and collaboration between the otolaryngologist and anesthesiologist are critical for providing quality acute pain management.

REFERENCES

1. Apfelbaum JL, Chen C, Mehta SS, et al. Postoperative pain experience: results from a national survey suggest postoperative pain continues to be undermanaged. Anesth Analg 2003;97(2):534–40. Available at: http://www.ncbi.nlm.nih.gov/pubmed/12873949. Accessed January 30, 2019.
2. Gan TJ, Habib AS, Miller TE, et al. Incidence, patient satisfaction, and perceptions of post-surgical pain: results from a US national survey. Curr Med Res Opin 2014;30(1):149–60.
3. Tighe P, Buckenmaier CC, Boezaart AP, et al. Acute pain medicine in the United States: a status report. Pain Med 2015;16(9):1806–26.
4. Alam A, Juurlink DN. The prescription opioid epidemic: an overview for anesthesiologists. Can J Anaesth 2016;63(1):61 8.
5. Cramer JD, Wisler B, Gouveia CJ. Opioid stewardship in otolaryngology: state of the art review. Otolaryngol Head Neck Surg 2018;158(5):817–27.
6. Kehlet H, Dahl JB. The value of "multimodal" or "balanced analgesia" in postoperative pain treatment. Anesth Analg 1993;77(5):1048–56. Available at: http://www.ncbi.nlm.nih.gov/pubmed/8105724. Accessed January 30, 2019.
7. Sun EC, Darnall BD, Baker LC, et al. Incidence of and risk factors for chronic opioid use among opioid-naive patients in the postoperative period. JAMA Intern Med 2016;176(9):1286–93.

8. Vadivelu N, Mitra S, Schermer E, et al. Preventive analgesia for postoperative pain control: a broader concept. Local Reg Anesth 2014;7:17–22.

9. American Society of Anesthesiologists Task Force on Acute Pain Management. Practice guidelines for acute pain management in the perioperative setting: an updated report by the American Society of Anesthesiologists Task Force on Acute Pain Management. Anesthesiology 2012;116(2):248–73.

10. Young AC, Buvanendran A. Multimodal analgesia: pharmacologic interventions and prevention of persistent postoperative pain. In: Hadzic A, editor. Hadzic's textbook of regional anesthesia and acute pain medicine. 2nd edition. New York: McGraw Hill; 2017. p. 1219–25.

11. Vane JR, Botting RM. Mechanism of action of anti-inflammatory drugs. Scand J Rheumatol 1996;25(sup102):9–21.

12. Southworth S, Peters J, Rock A, et al. A multicenter, randomized, double-blind, placebo- controlled trial of intravenous ibuprofen 400 and 800 mg every 6 hours in the management of postoperative pain. Clin Ther 2009;31(9):1922–35.

13. De Oliveira GS, Agarwal D, Benzon HT. Perioperative single dose ketorolac to prevent postoperative pain: a meta-analysis of randomized trials. Anesth Analg 2012;114(2):424–33.

14. Martinez V, Beloeil H, Marret E, et al. Non-opioid analgesics in adults after major surgery: systematic review with network meta-analysis of randomized trials. Br J Anaesth 2017;118(1):22–31.

15. Kelly LE, Sommer DD, Ramakrishna J, et al. Morphine or ibuprofen for post tonsillectomy analgesia: a randomized trial. Pediatrics 2015;135(2):307–13.

16. Moss JR, Watcha MF, Bendel LP, et al. A multicenter, randomized, double-blind placebo-controlled, single dose trial of the safety and efficacy of intravenous ibuprofen for treatment of pain in pediatric patients undergoing tonsillectomy. Paediatr Anaesth 2014;24(5):483–9.

17. Katz J. NSAIDs and COX-2 selective inhibitors. In: Benzon H, Raja S, Molloy R, editors. Essentials of pain medicine and regional anesthesia. 2nd edition; 2005. p. 141–58. Philadelphia: Elsevier.

18. Moeller C, Pawlowski J, Pappas AL, et al. The safety and efficacy of intravenous ketorolac in patients undergoing primary endoscopic sinus surgery: a randomized, double-blinded clinical trial. Int Forum Allergy Rhinol 2012;2(4):342–7.

19. Chin CJ, Franklin JH, Turner B, et al. Ketorolac in thyroid surgery: quantifying the risk of hematoma. J Otolaryngol Head Neck Surg 2011;40(3):196–9. Available at: http://www.ncbi.nlm.nih.gov/pubmed/21518639. Accessed February 20, 2019.

20. Jeyakumar A, Brickman TM, Williamson ME, et al. Nonsteroidal anti-inflammatory drugs and postoperative bleeding following adenotonsillectomy in pediatric patients. Arch Otolaryngol Head Neck Surg 2008;134(1):24.

21. Issioui T, Klein KW, White PF, et al. The efficacy of premedication with celecoxib and acetaminophen in preventing pain after otolaryngologic surgery. Anesth Analg 2002;94(5):1188–93.

22. Carpenter PS, Shepherd HM, McCrary H, et al. Association of celecoxib use with decreased opioid requirements after head and neck cancer surgery with free tissue reconstruction. JAMA Otolaryngol Head Neck Surg 2018;144(11):988–94.

23. Graham GG, Scott KF. Mechanism of action of paracetamol. Am J Ther 2005;12(1):46–55. Available at: http://www.ncbi.nlm.nih.gov/pubmed/15662292. Accessed February 20, 2019.

24. Romej M, Voepel-Lewis T, Merkel SI, et al. Effect of preemptive acetaminophen on postoperative pain scores and oral fluid intake in pediatric tonsillectomy patients.

AANA J 1996;64(6):535–40. Available at: http://www.ncbi.nlm.nih.gov/pubmed/9204788. Accessed February 20, 2019.

25. Remy C, Marret E, Bonnet F. State of the art of paracetamol in acute pain therapy. Curr Opin Anaesthesiol 2006;19(5):562–5.

26. Food and Drug Administration, HHS. Organ-specific warnings; internal analgesic, antipyretic, and antirheumatic drug products for over-the-counter human use; final monograph. Final rule. Fed Regist 2009;74(81):19385–409. Available at: http://www.ncbi.nlm.nih.gov/pubmed/19507324. Accessed February 20, 2019.

27. Larson AM, Polson J, Fontana RJ, et al. Acetaminophen-induced acute liver failure: results of a United States multicenter, prospective study. Hepatology 2005; 42(6):1364–72.

28. Spanknebel K, Chabot JA, DiGiorgi M, et al. Thyroidectomy using local anesthesia: a report of 1,025 cases over 16 years. J Am Coll Surg 2005;201(3): 375–85.

29. Khelemsky Y. Acute and chronic pain management. In: Levine AI, Govindaraj S, DeMaria Jr S, editors. Anesthesiology and otolaryngology. 1st edition. New York: Springer; 2013. p. 373–91.

30. Higashizawa T, Koga Y. Effect of infraorbital nerve block under general anesthesia on consumption of isoflurane and postoperative pain in endoscopic endonasal maxillary sinus surgery. J Anesth 2001;15(3):136–8.

31. DeMaria S, Govindaraj S, Chinosorvatana N, et al. Bilateral sphenopalatine ganglion blockade improves postoperative analgesia after endoscopic sinus surgery. Am J Rhinol Allergy 2012;26(1):e23–7.

32. Andreae MH, Andreae DA. Regional anaesthesia to prevent chronic pain after surgery: a cochrane systematic review and meta-analysis. Br J Anaesth 2013; 111(5):711–20.

33. Fassoulaki A, Triga A, Melemeni A, et al. Multimodal analgesia with gabapentin and local anesthetics prevents acute and chronic pain after breast surgery for cancer. Anesth Analg 2005;101(5):1427–32.

34. Butterworth JF, Strichartz GR. Molecular mechanisms of local anesthesia: a review. Anesthesiology 1990;72(4):711–34. Available at: http://www.ncbi.nlm.nih.gov/pubmed/2157353. Accessed February 27, 2019.

35. Butterworth J. Clinical pharmacology of local anesthetics. In: Hadzic A, editor. Hadzic's textbook of regional anesthesia and acute pain medicine. 2nd edition. New York: McGraw Hill; 2017. p. 124–37.

36. Chahar P, Cummings KC III. Liposomal bupivacaine: a review of a new bupivacaine formulation. J Pain Res 2012;5:257–64.

37. Sim AJ, Levine AI, Govindaraj S. Functional nasal and sinus surgery. In: Levine AI, Govindaraj S, DeMaria Jr S, editors. Anesthesiology and otolaryngology. 1st edition. New York: Springer; 2013. p. 197–216.

38. Pehora C, Pearson AM, Kaushal A, et al. Dexamethasone as an adjuvant to peripheral nerve block. Cochrane Database Syst Rev 2017;(11).CD011770.

39. Butterworth JF, Strichartz GR. The alpha 2-adrenergic agonists clonidine and guanfacine produce tonic and phasic block of conduction in rat sciatic nerve fibers. Anesth Analg 1993;76(2):295–301. Available at: http://www.ncbi.nlm.nih.gov/pubmed/8093828. Accessed February 27, 2019.

40. Eisenach JC, Gebhart GF. Intrathecal amitriptyline: antinociceptive interactions with intravenous morphine and intrathecal clonidine, neostigmine, and carbamylcholine in rats. Anesthesiology 1995;83:1036–45. Available at: http://anesthesiology.pubs.asahq.org/article.aspx?articleid=2323515. Accessed February 27, 2019.

41. Giordano D, Panini A, Pernice C, et al. Neurologic toxicity of lidocaine during awake intubation in a patient with tongue base abscess. Case report. Am J Otolaryngol 2014;35(1):62–5.

42. Neal JM, Bernards CM, Butterworth JF, et al. ASRA practice advisory on local anesthetic systemic toxicity. Reg Anesth Pain Med 2010;35(2):152–61.

43. Ogle OE, Mahjoubi G. Local anesthesia: agents, techniques, and complications. Dent Clin North Am 2012;56(1):133–48, ix.

44. Sola C, Dadure C, Choquet O, et al. Nerve blocks of the face. In: Hadzic A, editor. Hadzic's textbook of regional anesthesia and acute pain medicine. 2nd edition. New York: McGraw Hill; 2017. 535–51.

45. Tiippana EM, Hamunen K, Kontinen VK, et al. Do surgical patients benefit from perioperative gabapentin/pregabalin? A systematic review of efficacy and safety. Anesth Analg 2007;104(6):1545–56.

46. Hah J, Mackey SC, Schmidt P, et al. Effect of perioperative gabapentin on postoperative pain resolution and opioid cessation in a mixed surgical cohort: a randomized clinical trial. JAMA Surg 2018;153(4):303–11.

47. Amin S, Amr Y. Comparison between preemptive gabapentin and paracetamol for pain control after adenotonsillectomy in children. Anesth Essays Res 2011; 5(2):167.

48. Sanders JG, Dawes PJD. Gabapentin for perioperative analgesia in otorhinolaryngology–head and neck surgery. Otolaryngol Head Neck Surg 2016;155(6):893–903.

49. De Oliveira GS, Almeida MD, Benzon HT, et al. Perioperative single dose systemic dexamethasone for postoperative pain: a meta-analysis of randomized controlled trials. Anesthesiology 2011;115(3):575–88.

50. Diakos EA, Gallos ID, El-Shunnar S, et al. Dexamethasone reduces pain, vomiting and overall complications following tonsillectomy in adults: a systematic review and meta-analysis of randomised controlled trials. Clin Otolaryngol 2011;36(6): 531–42.

51. Afman CE, Welge JA, Steward DL. Steroids for post-tonsillectomy pain reduction: meta-analysis of randomized controlled trials. Otolaryngol Head Neck Surg 2006; 134(2):181–6.

52. Loftus RW, Yeager MP, Clark JA, et al. Intraoperative ketamine reduces perioperative opiate consumption in opiate-dependent patients with chronic back pain undergoing back surgery. Anesthesiology 2010;113(3):1.

53. Dahmani S, Michelet D, Abback P-S, et al. Ketamine for perioperative pain management in children: a meta-analysis of published studies. Paediatr Anaesth 2011;21(6):636–52.

54. Damghani MA, Haghbin MA, Karbasi E. The analgesic effects of ketamine, ketorolac and dexamethasone after adenotonsillectomy surgery in children aged 4 to 18 years. 2018;25. Available at: http://jkmu.kmu.ac.ir/article_76875_b9524406b5fc3d328c6e7eb4cd0cd632.pdf. Accessed February 27, 2019.

55. Tekelioglu UY, Apuhan T, Akkaya A, et al. Comparison of topical tramadol and ketamine in pain treatment after tonsillectomy. Paediatr Anaesth 2013;23(6): 496–501.

56. Allen CA, Ivester JR. Ketamine for pain management—side effects & potential adverse events. Pain Manag Nurs 2017;18(6):372–7.

57. Hanna MN, Ahmed O, Hall S. Intravenous patient-controlled analgesia. In: Hadzic A, editor. Hadzic's textbook of regional anesthesia and acute pain medicine. 2nd edition. New York: McGraw Hill; 2017. p. 1167–79.

58. Khonsary SA, Ma Q, Villablanca P, et al. Clinical functional anatomy of the pterygopalatine ganglion, cephalgia and related dysautonomias: a review. Surg Neurol Int 2013;4(Suppl 6):S422-8.
59. Chan BJ, Koushan K, Liszauer A, et al. Iatrogenic globe penetration in a case of infraorbital nerve block. Can J Ophthalmol 2011;46(3):290-1.
60. Abubaker AK, Al-Qudah MA. The role of endoscopic sphenopalatine ganglion block on nausea and vomiting after sinus surgery. Am J Rhinol Allergy 2018; 32(5):369-73.
61. Preziosi BD, Hershkin AT, Seider PJ, et al. Oral & maxillofacial regional anesthesia. In: Hadzic A, editor. Hadzic's textbook of regional anesthesia and acute pain medicine. 2nd edition. New York: McGraw Hill; 2017. p. 662-81.
62. Bendtsen TF, Abbas S, Chan V. Ultrasound-guided cervical plexus block. In: Hadzic A, editor. Hadzic's textbook of regional anesthesia and acute pain medicine. 2nd edition. New York: McGraw Hill; 2017. p. 552-7.
63. Ahmad I. Regional and topical anesthesia for awake endotracheal intubation. In: Hadzic A, editor. Hadzic's textbook of regional anesthesia and acute pain medicine. 2nd edition. New York: McGraw Hill; 2017. p. 289-99.

Anesthesia and Chronic Pain Management

Anuj Malhotra, MD[a], Mourad Shehebar, MD[a], Yury Khelemsky, MD[a,b],*

KEYWORDS

- Chronic pain • Postoperative pain • Anesthesia

KEY POINTS

- Severe acute postoperative pain is the biggest predictor of chronic postsurgical pain.
- Chronic head and neck pain can be nociceptive, neuropathic, or both.
- Interventional approaches can help diagnose and treat pain and decrease the need for medications.
- Opioids may be appropriate for postoperative and for cancer pain, but other medications have better efficacy and safety profiles in nonmalignant pain syndromes.
- A multidisciplinary team approach can be helpful in diagnosing and treating complex pain syndromes.

INTRODUCTION

The reasons for development of chronic pain are complex and poorly understood.[1] Its emergence stems from an aberrant physiologic response to surgery or disease-state, as well as other patient-related and environmental factors. Genetic factors likely play an important role in predicting who will develop chronic pain.[1]

Over 20% of adults in the United States have chronic pain, with 8% having high-impact chronic pain. The burden of chronic pain after treatment of major head and neck malignancy has been reported in approximately 1 in 3 patients.[2] The lack of long-term efficacy of opioids in the treatment of chronic pain, coupled with the inherent risks of these compounds, as witnessed by the current opioid crisis, necessitates the development of comprehensive multimodal approaches to better treat persistent pain conditions.[3]

Disclosure Statement: Dr A. Malhotra and Dr M. Shehebar have nothing to disclose. Dr Y. Khelemsky is on the Advisory Board for Averitas Pharmaceuticals.
[a] Department of Anesthesiology, Perioperative and Pain Medicine, Icahn School of Medicine at Mount Sinai, One Gustave L. Levy Place, KCC 8th Floor, Box 1010, New York, NY 10029, USA; [b] Department of Neurology, Icahn School of Medicine at Mount Sinai, One Gustave L. Levy Place, KCC 8th Floor, Box 1010, New York, NY 10029, USA
* Corresponding author. Department of Anesthesiology, Perioperative and Pain Medicine, Icahn School of Medicine at Mount Sinai, One Gustave L. Levy Place, KCC 8th Floor, Box 1010, New York, NY 10029.
E-mail address: Yury.khelemsky@mountsinai.org

Otolaryngol Clin N Am 52 (2019) 1083–1094
https://doi.org/10.1016/j.otc.2019.08.007
0030-6665/19/© 2019 Elsevier Inc. All rights reserved.

PAIN DEFINITION: THE INTERNATIONAL ASSOCIATION FOR THE STUDY OF PAIN

The International Association for the Study of Pain (IASP) defines pain as "an unpleasant sensory and emotional experience associated with actual or potential tissue damage, or described in terms of such damage."[4] It is, therefore, important for practitioners to understand that pain is not simply the summation of nociceptive input, but rather a patient's experience of that input.

CHRONIC PAIN DEFINITION, INCIDENCE OF CHRONIC POSTSURGICAL PAIN

Chronic pain, typically defined as lasting more than 3 months and/or when such pain lasts longer than the anticipated healing time.[4] Chronic postsurgical pain (CPSP) is described as pain that is present after surgery, with other etiologies ruled out (including exacerbation of pre-existing conditions), and greater than 2 months in duration.[5,6]

CPSP is multifactorial, as it may have physical, psychological, genetic, and social inputs.[7] It has been shown that multiple surgical procedures within the same peripheral nerve distribution increase the risk of CPSP.[8] Incidence varies widely dependent on surgical site, clinical level of care, and even study design. A known consistent risk factor in developing CPSP is severe acute postoperative pain.[8]

Incisional pain and neuropathic pain are leading causes of CPSP.[9] These usually stem from an intraoperative nerve injury.[10,11] Both mechanically induced neuropathy and inflammatory immunologic components may have a role. Postsurgical inflammatory neuropathy has been confirmed via nerve biopsies in a subset of patients regardless of the existence of mechanical injury.[12] Nerve blocks placed perioperatively for procedures that are known to cause severe postoperative pain may be able to mitigate the formation of CPSP.[13,14]

TYPES OF PAIN: NEUROPATHIC, NOCICEPTIVE

Fundamentally, pain can be classified into nociceptive and neuropathic pain. Nociceptive pain has an identifiable etiology caused by tissue damage from direct activation of pain nerve fibers, either due to chemical, inflammatory, or mechanical mediators.

Nociceptive pain can be further divided into somatic and visceral pain. Somatic pain is well localized and is described as sharp or throbbing. Visceral pain is usually characterized as dull and more difficult to locate precisely. Neuropathic pain refers to pain that is a result of either central nervous system or peripheral nerve dysfunction or lesion.[15] Neuropathic pain may be caused by explicit injury to large nerve structures or by presumed damage to minor peripheral nerve structures. This pain tends to be described as burning, tingling, or lancinating in nature. Chronic neuropathic pain is the most common type of CPSP and intuitively is the type of pain most refractory to treatment.[16]

PAIN TRANSMISSION

Nociceptive signals from the periphery are transmitted via C fibers (unmyelinated small axons with slow conduction) and A-delta fibers (lightly myelinated axons with rapid conduction). Spinal neurons receiving cutaneous thermal and pain input are located primarily in (Rexed) laminae I and II, while those receiving mechanical information are located in laminae IV and V. Visceral input is received by neurons in laminae III, VII, and X. The substantia gelatinosa (laminae II), which contains a high concentration of opioid receptors, plays a vital role in modulation and mediation of pain perception. Cutaneous nociceptive information is conducted to the thalamus mainly via spinothalamic pathway, whereas visceral nociceptive input is conducted via postsynaptic dorsal column pathway. The ventral posterolateral nucleus of the thalamus offers site-specific information to the somatosensory cortex. Other thalamic nuclei relay nociceptive input to cingulate cortices, which create affective responses to pain. Descending modulation of input adds another level of complexity to nociceptive signal transduction. Wide dynamic range (WDR) neurons are found in the dorsal horn of the spinal cord and are involved in wind-up. Wind-up can intensify responses of dorsal horn neurons by up to 20-fold and prolong responses even after the initial peripheral input cessation, which generates central hypersensitivity.[17]

PERTINENT ANATOMY

In regard to head and neck sensation, the cell bodies of trigeminal sensory neurons are situated in the trigeminal sensory ganglion, which corresponds to dorsal root ganglion. The second-order neurons in the trigeminothalamic pathway are located in the chief sensory nucleus of the trigeminal nerve, which is in the pons. These fibers cross midline and ascend to the thalamus in the trigeminal lemniscus. Additionally, these axons terminate in the ventral posterior nucleus of the thalamus, medial to those from the limbs and trunk. Third-order thalamocortical neurons synapse at the primary somatosensory cortex. Information from the oral cavity travels to the ipsilateral thalamus via the dorsal trigeminothalamic tract.

Pain and temperature fibers also have cell bodies in the trigeminal ganglion. The central processes enter the pons via the trigeminal nerve root and descend to synapse in the spinal nucleus of the trigeminal nerve, which is similar to the substantia gelatinosa. Axons arising from second-order neurons cross midline to join the trigeminal lemniscus also known as the trigeminothalamic tract. The A-delta fibers terminate in the ventroposteromedial (VPM) thalamus, whereas the C-fibers terminate in the parafasciculus (PF) and centromedian (CM) thalamus. The axons then synapse on the primary somatosensory cortex. The trigeminal lemniscus of the head is functionally analogous to both the dorsal column medial lemniscus and spinothalamic systems of the body.

TRIGEMINAL NERVE

The trigeminal nerve, the fifth cranial nerve (CN V), is the most complex and largest of the 12 cranial nerves and has an extensive anatomic course. It provides motor innervation for muscles of mastication as well as sensation to the face, oral and nasal cavities, and most of the scalp. The trigeminal nerve trifurcates into the ophthalmic (V1), maxillary (V2), and mandibular (V3) nerves distal to the trigeminal (eg, gasserian) ganglion, which is located within Meckel cave.[18]

The ophthalmic nerve passes through the orbit superiorly and then re-enters the frontal bone briefly before exiting above the orbit through the superior orbital fissure. The ophthalmic nerve provides sensation to the eye, lachrymal glands, conjunctiva, part of the nasal mucosa, as well as skin of the nose, eyelid, and forehead.

The maxillary branch exits the skull through the foramen rotundum, inferolateral to the cavernous sinus. It then passes through the pterygopalatine fossa, where it gives off several branches. The main branch continues anteriorly in the orbital floor and materializes onto the face as the infraorbital nerve to innervate the middle third of the face and upper teeth.

The mandibular nerve typically runs laterally along the skull base, then exits the cranium by descending through the foramen ovale and provides sensation to the lower third of the face, tongue, floor of the mouth, and jaw. The motor component innervates 4muscles of mastication.

GLOSSOPHARYNGEAL NERVE

Cranial nerve IX, also known as the glossopharyngeal nerve, is a mixed nerve that carries both afferent sensory and efferent motor information. It exits the brainstem from the upper medulla and leaves the skull through the jugular foramen. It then descends beneath the styloid process and penetrates the pharyngeal constrictor muscle, which reaches the posterior tongue and terminates in several branches that provide sensation to the

Oropharynx
Carotid body/sinus
Posterior third of the tongue (along with taste)
Middle ear cavity and parasympathetic innervation of the parotid gland
Motor innervation of the stylopharyngeus muscle of the pharynx

SPHENOPALATINE GANGLION

The sphenopalatine ganglion (SPG) is a mostly parasympathetic ganglion, primarily fed by the greater petrosal nerve (branch of facial nerve), found in the pterygopalatine fossa, and contains the largest collection of neurons outside the brain.[19] It receives sensory, parasympathetic, and sympathetic inputs. The axons of the SPG project to the lacrimal glands, nasal mucosa, hard palate, gingiva, and mucosa of buccal cavity, and control blood flow to the area.

SUPERFICIAL CERVICAL PLEXUS AND DEEP CERVICAL PLEXUS

The cervical plexus is formed by the anterior rami of the first 4 cervical spinal nerves. This plexus is located lateral to the transverse processes between prevertebral muscles and posterior to the sternocleidomastoid. It gives off 2 branches, the superficial and deep plexus. The superficial branch supplies skin of the anterolateral neck and scalp via transverse cervical and lesser occipital nerve, outer ear via great auricular nerve, and skin above and below the clavicle via supraclavicular nerve.

The deep cervical plexus consists of the looped ansa cervicalis (C1-3), providing innervation to the anterior neck muscles, as well as giving various branches to posterolateral neck muscles. Additionally, the phrenic nerve, which innervates the diaphragm and pericardium, can also be attributed to the deep cervical plexus.

BRACHIAL PLEXUS

The brachial plexus is a network of somatic nerves formed by the ventral rami of cervical spinal nerves (C5-T1). It provides afferent and efferent nerve fibers to the chest, shoulder, arm, and hand. This plexus stretches from the spinal cord through the cervicoaxillary canal in the neck, over the first rib, and into the axilla. The plexus is primarily responsible for the motor innervation of all the muscles in the upper extremity with the exception of the trapezius and levator scapula.[20] It also supplies all the cutaneous innervation of the upper limb with the exception of the axilla (supplied by supraclavicular nerve) and the dorsal scapula area (supplied by cutaneous branches of the dorsal rami). The plexus is divided into roots, trunks, divisions, cords, and branches.

OCCIPITAL NERVES

The greater occipital nerve (GON) arises from the medial branch of the dorsal primary ramus of second cervical nerve. The GON, along with the occipital artery, penetrates the fascia below the superior nuchal ridge and supplies innervation to the medial portion of the posterior scalp.

The lesser occipital nerve (LON) is supplied by the lateral branch of ventral rami of the second and third cervical nerves. The LON travels superiorly along the posterior aspect of the sternocleidomastoid muscle, branching into cutaneous innervation of the lateral posterior scalp and cranial surface of the pinna.

CERVICAL SPINE

The cervical spine consists of 7 vertebrae, of which the upper 2 (C1 and C2, the atlas and axis, respectively) are distinct from the lower 5. C3-6 vertebra has a flattened body and triangular vertebral foramina. The facet joints are diarthrodial synovial joints with fibrous capsules. These joints are innervated by both anterior and posterior rami. The atlanto-occipital and atlantoaxial joints are innervated by the anterior rami of the first and second cervical spinal nerves, whereas C2-3 is innervated by the 2 branches of the posterior ramus of the third cervical spinal nerve, the third occipital nerve. The remaining facets are innervated by the posterior rami of the medial branches that arise 1 level cephalad and caudad to the joint. These medial branches send articular branches to the facet joints as they wrap around the waists of the articular pillars.[21]

Exiting at each vertebral level is a spinal nerve, which is the union of the anterior and posterior nerve roots. The spinal nerve typically occupies about 25% of the foraminal space. It's bordered superiorly by the pedicle of the previously mentioned vertebrae, inferiorly by the lower pedicle, posterolaterally by facet joints, and anteromedially by the uncovertebral joints. These nerves exit above the corresponding numbered vertebral body from C2-7; thus the C3 nerve root exits via the C2/3 neural foramen.

CHRONIC PAIN SYNDROMES OF HEAD AND NECK

Chronic pain of the head and neck can occur as the result of primary malignancy with compressive or infiltrative effects on a nerve or plexus.[22] It can also occur as the sequela of surgical resection or manipulation, either from direct nerve ligation, injury from retraction or prolonged stretch, entrapment in scar, formation of neuroma, or from myalgia caused by denervation or resection of muscle. Radiation injury can result in plexopathy or dystonia,[23] while chemotherapy may result in more diffuse neuropathic pain. Given the dense innervation of the head and neck, multiple pain syndromes may be present in the same patient. Careful history and physical examination, provocative maneuvers, and testing of sensory fields can give an initial clue to diagnosis. This is often followed by diagnostic injections, followed by repeated therapeutic injections if response is confirmed, and sometimes neuromodulatory or ablative techniques. Often direct interventional techniques are supplemented by use of appropriate medication management, with a focus on antineuropathic agents, muscle relaxants, and topical agents.[24] Special consideration should be given to mode of delivery in this patient population if oral intake is limited, as not all formulations can be crushed and administered via a feeding tube.[25]

Another consideration with head and neck pain is exacerbation of chronic, nonmalignant pain. This can be from worsened biomechanics, increased axial loading, medication overuse, and exacerbation of underlying headaches.[26] Practitioners should be alerted to this possibility, particularly if symptoms predate diagnosis or treatment of malignancy, if symptoms more closely mimic nonmalignant pain states, or if symptoms manifest well after treatment has been completed.

With head and neck cancer, at least 50% of patients experience significant pain, while 10% report severe pain.[27] Pain should properly be evaluated, monitored, and managed during routine follow-up.[27] During the first year of diagnosis of malignancy, many patients are diagnosed with a comorbid mood disorder (eg, anxiety or depression), which should be appropriately addressed to effectively assist in treating cancer-related pain.[28]

SPECIFIC CHRONIC PAIN SYNDROMES
Chronic Postsurgical Pain

Chronic postsurgical pain (CPSP) is defined by the International Association for the Study of Pain as postoperative pain lasting longer than 2 months in the absence of ongoing tissue injury and in the absence of preoperative pain.[29] Risk factors for CPSP are described across many types of surgery and frequently include emergent surgery, reoperation, depression, surgical wound complication, female gender, pre-existing chronic pain, and persistent acute pain. Incidence is variable, ranging from less than 5% in low-risk surgeries to as high as 25% to 65%.[30] Generally, the more highly innervated the area operated on and the more invasive the surgery, the higher the frequency and intensity of CPSP will be, with thoracotomy, mastectomy, and inguinal herniorraphy having the highest reported rates. Certain types of head and neck surgery would be expected to have a high incidence of CPSP, although quantification is challenging because of significant variability in procedures.[8]

Common causes of CPSP are scar entrapment and neuroma formation.[31] These manifest as neuropathic pain, with onset several weeks to months after surgery as the affected nerve becomes adherent in scar tissue or a neuroma forms from injured nerves. Often patients will report a focal point from which the pain radiates, which can be in the scar itself or in muscle layers below. Replication of usual pain with light pressure or tapping over the area is referred to as a Tinel sign and often, sensory hyper- or hypoesthesia will be present in a nearby nerve's distribution. Scar injection with local anesthetic with or without steroid can be diagnostic and therapeutic. Ultrasound guidance can be helpful if deeper neuromas are suspected, both for enhanced accuracy and safety. Neuromodulation or neurolysis of neuromas can be performed using phenol, alcohol, radiofrequency, cryoablation, pulsed radiofrequency, peripheral stimulator implant, or surgical neurectomy.[32]

Trigeminal Neuralgia

Trigeminal neuralgia (TN) occurs as paroxysmal, lancinating pain in 1 or all distributions of the trigeminal nerve, lasting seconds at a time. The pain is often the result of vascular compression of the exiting cranial nerve V at the brainstem and may be amenable to surgical decompression in these cases.[33] Entrapment or injury to branches of the trigeminal nerve may also occur, and nerve blocks can be performed using fluoroscopic or ultrasound guidance to access the Gasserian ganglion via the foramen ovale or V2 and V3 at the lateral pterygoid plate via a subzygomatic approach. Repeat local anesthetic blockade, addition of steroid, neuromodulation (eg, pulsed radiofrequency or cryotherapy), or ablative techniques (eg, radiofrequency ablation or gamma knife) can also be of benefit.[34] It should be noted that 5% of patients with multiple sclerosis experience an episode of TN, so this diagnosis should be considered in the work-up of TN.

Glossopharyngeal Neuralgia

Glossopharyngeal neuralgia produces a distinct neuropathic pain along the sensory distribution of cranial nerve IX, which consists of the posterior tongue and pharynx, as well as parts of the ear canal and tympanic membrane. Pain is often described as "shooting out the ear." Eagle syndrome is form of glossopharyngeal neuralgia caused by an elongated styloid process causing pressure on the nerve, and may be accompanied by vascular manifestations if there is pressure on the carotid artery.[35] Ultrasound-guided injection can aid in the diagnosis, but the ultimate treatment is a surgical styloidectomy.

Atypical Facial Pain

Persistent idiopathic facial pain (PIFP) refers to pain along the territory of the trigeminal nerve that does not fit the classic presentation of other cranial neuralgias or headache syndromes.[36] The pain is usually constant and may or may not have neuropathic features. Peripheral nerve blocks of the terminal trigeminal branches such as the supraorbital, infraorbital, and mandibular may be of benefit if the pain is well localized. Sphenopalatine block in the pterygopalatine fossa may be performed via intraoral, transnasal, or percutaneous approaches and can be helpful if midface pain or autonomic symptoms are present.

Cervical Dystonia

Dystonia is defined by involuntary spasm, repetitive motion, and increased tone with loss of normal range. It may be constant or worsened with activity. Causes include genetic variants, trauma, and idiopathic response to neuroleptic medications. Specific dystonias of the head and neck include torticollis, spasmodic dysphonia, and blepharospasm. Interventional treatment includes physical therapy, distraction-based techniques, injection of botulinum toxin, and deep-brain stimulation.[37]

Thoracic Outlet Syndrome

Thoracic outlet syndrome can manifest as vascular compression (arterial or venous), brachial plexopathy, or both.[38,39] Diagnosis includes physical examination testing (Roos, Adson) and imaging (computed tomography [CT] angiogram, MRI neurogram), as well as ruling out more common pain syndromes. Symptoms are positional and replicable, usually resolving completely between episodes. Entrapment can occur in the interscalene groove, as the plexus passes between the clavicle and T1 rib (or C7 rib, if present), or in the subpectoralis minor space as the brachial plexus, subclavian artery, and vein enter the axilla. Treatment includes physical therapy, botulinum toxin injection of the scalene muscles, or surgical resection.

Occipital Neuralgia

Occipital neuralgia can refer to neuropathic pain in the head in the distribution of the greater (medial and posterior), lesser (lateral), or third (thin medial stripe) occipital nerves. These nerves arise from the primary posterior ramus of C2 in the case of greater and lesser, and the medial branches of C2-3 in the case of the third occipital nerve. Multiple entrapment sites are possible, including at the intersection of the semispinalis capitis and obliquus capitis inferior, the trapezius insertion on scalp, and at the C2-3 facet joint.[40] These nerves are often involved in whiplash injury given multiple flexion points they traverse within the musculoskeletal system of the neck. Palpation-based, ultrasound-guided, and fluoroscopic-guided nerve blocks, radiofrequency ablation, and peripheral nerve stimulators have been used with good effect.[41]

Postherpetic Neuralgia

Acute herpes zoster (eg, shingles) can occur in any branch of cranial nerve V (most commonly V1), in the facial nerve (Ramsay-Hunt syndrome), or in upper cervical dermatomes to produce neuropathic head and neck pain. Prompt diagnosis and treatment with antivirals are the mainstays of therapy. Involvement of V1 can be particularly concerning for sequelae including corneal scarring, uveitis, and vision loss.[42] Ramsay-Hunt syndrome can produce temporary facial paralysis. Interventional treatment may include steroid injection of the involved nerve. Postherpetic neuralgia (PHN) occurs when pain remains more than 3 months after an outbreak of shingles, and incidence is related to the severity of the acute presentation.

Cervical Radiculopathy

Cervical radicular pain can be caused by disc herniation or facet hypertrophy with resulting neuroforaminal stenosis. Impingement of the upper cervical nerve roots (typically C3 or C4) can result in neck and facial pain. Pain is ipsilateral and dermatomal, and may be provoked by Spurling maneuver. Most cases of cervical radicular pain are self-limited and may be managed conservatively. Epidural steroid injection via the interlaminar route has become the mainstay of therapy, with the transforaminal route falling out of favor because of the high incidence of intra-arterial injection within the foramen, occurring in up to 25% of injections.[43] Failure of conservative pain management or the presence of neurologic compromise may necessitate surgical intervention.

Cervical Spondylosis

Cervical facet arthropathy produces achy, axial neck pain worse with extension and turning. There may be radiation to the occiput, face, or shoulders, and there can be exacerbation of underlying headaches. Intra-articular facet injections are unreliable given the low volume of the joints and the potential for capsular disruption. Most practitioners instead perform diagnostic blockade of the medial branches that innervate the joints, after which radiofrequency ablation can be performed to yield longer-term relief.[44] Surgery is rarely indicated for this condition unless myelopathy is also present.

Temporomandibular Joint Disorders

Temporomandibular joint (TMJ) pain can radiate to the temple or neck and is worsened with chewing and talking. It can exacerbate underlying primary headache disorders. There may be associated bruxism, which should be suspected if the patient awakens with severe pain in the morning. In extreme cases, there can be disruption or dislocation of the TMJ disc, resulting in open or closed lock, necessitating manual reduction. Interventional approaches include use of a mouth guard, physical therapy, trigger point injections, botulinum toxin injection of the temporalis or masseter, steroid injection, or visco-supplementation of the joint.[45]

Medication Overuse Headache

Use of analgesics, particularly opioids, triptans, barbiturates, and nonsteroidal anti-inflammatory drugs (NSAIDs) for pain of the head and neck can cause worsening of underlying headaches, even if used to treat nonheadache pain.[26] Recommendations are to limit use of these medications to fewer than 7 to 10 days per month or to cease altogether, which often re-establishes the primary episodic headache that can then be treated.

CHRONIC PAIN MEDICATION MANAGEMENT

First-line treatment of acute or subacute head and neck pain, particularly if caused by injury or surgery, is conservative. Initial treatment is generally with as-needed analgesic dosing with the goal of taper to off as pain improves. NSAIDs inhibit cyclooxygenase (COX) 1 and 2, thereby decreasing inflammation and pain. Long-term use should be weighed against cardiac risk, specifically increased myocardial infarction (worse with COX 2-selective agents) or worsening congestive heart failure (worse with non-specific COX selective agents). Acetaminophen is thought to work centrally through inhibition of prostaglandin synthesis and is often used as an adjunct because of tolerability and good safety profile. Weak opioids or opioid-like medications (tramadol, tapentadol) may be indicated in the acute period if pain is severe, exerting their effects in the brain and dorsal horn of the spinal cord to inhibit ascending signals to the somatosensory cortex. These should be avoided for the long-term treatment of nonmalignant pain because of the development of tolerance, potential for opioid-induced hyperalgesia, and concerns for addiction or diversion.[46] Particular concern should be given to risk of respiratory depression in patients with head and neck pain who may have undergone operation predisposing to obstruction. Additionally, route of administration must be considered, as not all formulations can be crushed (eg, extended-release formulations) if the patient is unable to swallow pills. Such situations may necessitate use of transdermal (fentanyl, buprenorphine) or true long-acting opioids (methadone, buprenorphine) if indicated.

Antineuropathic agents should be considered early and should optimally precede opioid initiation, especially in the case of noncancer pain.[47] Local anesthetic creams or patches can be of particular use if a superficial source of pain is suspected, such as scar neuroma. Capsaicin creams act at the TRPV-1 receptor to peripherally deplete substance P and can decrease neuropathic pain with regular use; however, care must be taken to avoid mucous membranes, relevant when used for head and neck pain.

Gabapentinoids are often used because of minimal interaction with other medications and a favorable safety profile. Gabapentin and pregabalin act as modulators of calcium channels, found in abundance on small nerve terminals and in the dorsal horn of the spinal cord. They are dosed 2 to 3 times daily and require slow titration up to a therapeutic dose to allow for development of tolerance to the sedative side effects. Tricyclic antidepressants (TCAs) are also beneficial for treating neuropathic pain, with the lowest number needed to treat (NNT) of all antineuropathic medications[47] because of mechanisms of action including serotonin and norepinephrine reuptake inhibition, NMDA antagonism, and sodium channel blockade, among others. Second-generation TCAs such as nortriptyline and desipramine, the active metabolites of first-generation amitriptyline and imipramine, are often easier tolerated because of fewer sedating side effects. Selective norepinephrine receptor inhibitors such as venlafaxine and duloxetine have also been shown to improve neuropathic pain and are more likely to be of benefit than selective serotonin reuptake inhibitors. If these options are exhausted, anticonvulsants with sodium- or calcium channel-blocking properties such as topiramate, levetiracetam, and carbamazepine may be tried, although these agents require closer monitoring because of the potential for rare but serious adverse events (eg, hepatotoxicity and agranulocytosis). Carbamazepine and oxcarbazepine are of particular benefit for facial neuralgias and warrant an early trial if severe trigeminal neuralgia, glossopharyngeal neuralgia, or atypical facial pain is present. Memantine is an NMDA-receptor antagonist that can be of use if other antineuropathics are not tolerated because of sedation or falls risk, particularly relevant for use in the elderly population. Muscle relaxants including baclofen, cyclobenzaprine, and tizanidine are effective for treating spasm and dystonia.

SUMMARY

Chronic head and neck pain is often multifactorial owing to the overlapping innervation of closely located structures. Pain caused by malignancy may be due to the cancer itself or an adverse effect of treatment. Early, effective analgesia is most likely to limit progression to chronic pain. Identification and treatment of neuropathic pain with appropriate medications and interventional approaches when possible can significantly improve symptoms and limit reliance on breakthrough medication. Opioids may be appropriate in the short term for severe, acute pain and for evolving cancer pain; however, for nonmalignant pain, evidence is limited, and use of nonopioid adjuncts is favored.[48] Multiple specialties working together, including otolaryngology, neurology, neurosurgery, psychiatry, and pain management may be required in complex cases.

REFERENCES

1. Shipton EA. The transition from acute to chronic post surgical pain. Anaesth Intensive Care 2011;39(5):824–36.
2. Terkawi AS, Isang S, Alshehri AS, et al. The burden of chronic pain after major head and neck tumor therapy. Saudi J Anaesth 2017;11(Suppl 1):S71–9.
3. Marshall B, Bland MK, Hulla R, et al. Considerations in addressing the opioid epidemic and chronic pain within the USA. Pain Manag 2019;9(2):131–8.
4. McCain GA. Classification of chronic pain, edited by Harold Merskey and Nikolai Bogduk. J Musculoskelet Pain 1995;3(4):111–2.
5. Macrae WA. Chronic pain after surgery. Br J Anaesth 2001;87(1):88–98.
6. Gerbershagen HJ. Transition from acute to chronic postsurgical pain. Physiology, risk factors and prevention. Schmerz 2013;27(1):81–93 [quiz: 94–5]. [in German].
7. Hinrichs-Rocker A, Schulz K, Järvinen I, et al. Psychosocial predictors and correlates for chronic post-surgical pain (CPSP) - A systematic review. Eur J Pain 2009; 13(7):719–30.
8. Kehlet H, Jensen TS, Woolf CJ. Persistent postsurgical pain: risk factors and prevention. Lancet 2006;367(9522):1618–25.
9. Haroutiunian S, Nikolajsen L, Finnerup NB, et al. The neuropathic component in persistent postsurgical pain: a systematic literature review. Pain 2013;154(1): 95–102.
10. Callesen T, Bech K, Kehlet H. Prospective study of chronic pain after groin hernia repair. Br J Surg 1999;86(12):1528–31.
11. Benedetti F, Amanzio M, Casadio C, et al. Postoperative pain and superficial abdominal reflexes after posterolateral thoracotomy. Ann Thorac Surg 1997; 64(1):207–10.
12. Staff NP, Engelstad J, Klein CJ, et al. Post-surgical inflammatory neuropathy. Brain 2010;133(10):2866–80.
13. Obata H, Saito S, Fujita N, et al. Epidural block with mepivacaine before surgery reduces long-term post-thoracotomy pain. Can J Anaesth 1999;46(12):1127–32.
14. Andreae MH, Andreae DA. Local anaesthetics and regional anaesthesia for preventing chronic pain after surgery. Cochrane Database Syst Rev 2012;(10):CD007105.

15. Harden RN. Chronic neuropathic pain. Mechanisms, diagnosis, and treatment. Neurologist 2005;11(2):111–22.
16. Kanner R. Diagnosis and management of neuropathic pain in patients with cancer. Cancer Invest 2001;19(3):324–33.
17. Dickenson AH. Spinal cord pharmacology of pain. Br J Anaesth 1995;75(2): 193–200.
18. Kamel HA, Toland J. Trigeminal nerve anatomy: illustrated using examples of abnormalities. AJR Am J Roentgenol 2001;176(1):247–51.
19. Robbins MS, Robertson CE, Kaplan E, et al. The sphenopalatine ganglion: anatomy, pathophysiology, and therapeutic targeting in headache. Headache 2016; 56(2):240–58.
20. Leffert RD. Brachial-plexus injuries. N Engl J Med 1974;291(20):1059–67.
21. Bogduk N. The clinical anatomy of the cervical dorsal rami. Spine (Phila Pa 1976) 1982;7(4):319–30.
22. Marulli G, Battistella L, Mammana M, et al. Superior sulcus tumors (Pancoast tumors). Ann Transl Med 2016;4(12):239.
23. Epstein JB, Wilkie DJ, Fischer DJ, et al. Neuropathic and nociceptive pain in head and neck cancer patients receiving radiation therapy. Head Neck Oncol 2009;1:26.
24. Bianchini C, Malagò M, Crema L, et al. Post-operative pain management in head and neck cancer patients: predictive factors and efficacy of therapy. Acta Otorhinolaryngol Ital 2016;36(2):91–6.
25. Carmignani I, Locatello LG, Desideri I, et al. Analysis of dysphagia in advanced-stage head-and-neck cancer patients: impact on quality of life and development of a preventive swallowing treatment. Eur Arch Otorhinolaryngol 2018;275(8): 2159–67.
26. Diener HC, Holle D, Solbach K, et al. Medication-overuse headache: risk factors, pathophysiology and management. Nat Rev Neurol 2016;12(10):575–83.
27. Scharpf J, Karnell LH, Christensen AJ, et al. The role of pain in head and neck cancer recurrence and survivorship. Arch Otolaryngol Head Neck Surg 2009; 135(8):789–94.
28. Hammerlid E, Ahlner-Elmqvist M, Bjordal K, et al. A prospective multicentre study in Sweden and Norway of mental distress and psychiatric morbidity in head and neck cancer patients. Br J Cancer 1999;80(5–6):766–74.
29. Macrae WA. Chronic postsurgical pain. In: Crombie IK, LS, Croft P, et al, editors. Epidemiology of pain. 1999. p. 125–42. Seattle (WA).
30. Schug SA. Chronic pain after surgery or injury. Pain Clin Updates 2011;19(1):1–5.
31. Trescot AM, Karl HW. Nerve entrapment headaches at the temple: zygomatico-temporal and/or auriculotemporal nerve? Pain Physician 2019;22(1):E15–36.
32. Decrouy-Duruz V, Christen T, Raffoul W. Evaluation of surgical treatment for neuropathic pain from neuroma in patients with injured peripheral nerves. J Neurosurg 2018;128(4):1235–40.
33. Gandhoke GS, Smith KJ, Niranjan A, et al. Comparing microvascular decompression with gamma knife radiosurgery for trigeminal neuralgia a cost-effectiveness analysis. World Neurosurg 2019;125:207–16.
34. Wu H, Zhou J, Chen J, et al. Therapeutic efficacy and safety of radiofrequency ablation for the treatment of trigeminal neuralgia: a systematic review and meta-analysis. J Pain Res 2019;12:423–41.
35. Reddy GD, Viswanathan A. Trigeminal and glossopharyngeal neuralgia. Neurol Clin 2014;32(2):539–52.

36. Benoliel R, Gaul C. Persistent idiopathic facial pain. Cephalalgia 2017;37(7): 680–91.
37. Tatu LJW. Persistent idiopathic facial pain: "Dysfunction follows form". J Neural Transm 2017;124(2):237–43.
38. Ferrante MA, Ferrante ND. The thoracic outlet syndromes: Part 1. Overview of the thoracic outlet syndromes and review of true neurogenic thoracic outlet syndrome. Muscle Nerve 2017;55(6):782–93.
39. Ferrante MA, Ferrante ND. The thoracic outlet syndromes: Part 2. The arterial, venous, neurovascular, and disputed thoracic outlet syndromes. Muscle Nerve 2017;56(4):663–73.
40. Narouze S. Occipital neuralgia diagnosis and treatment: the role of ultrasound. Headache 2016;56(4):801–7.
41. Rodrigo D, Acin P, Bermejo P. Occipital nerve stimulation for refractory chronic migraine: results of a long-term prospective study. Pain Physician 2017;20(1): E151–9.
42. Vrcek ICE, Durairaj V. Herpes zoster ophthalmicus: a review for the internist. Am J Med 2017;130(1):21–6.
43. Schneider BJ, Maybin S, Sturos E. Safety and complications of cervical epidural steroid injections. Phys Med Rehabil Clin N Am 2018;29(1):155–69.
44. Golovac S. Radiofrequency neurolysis. Neuroimaging Clin N Am 2010;20(2): 203–14.
45. Moldez MA, Camones VR, Ramos GE, et al. Effectiveness of Intra-articular injections of sodium hyaluronate or corticosteroids for intracapsular temporomandibular disorders: a systematic review and meta-analysis. J Oral Facial Pain Headache 2018;32(1):53–66.
46. McDermott JD, Eguchi M, Stokes WA, et al. Short- and long-term opioid use in patients with oral and oropharynx cancer. Otolaryngol Head Neck Surg 2018; 160(3):409–19.
47. Clark GT, Padilla M, Dionne R. Medication treatment efficacy and chronic orofacial pain. Oral Maxillofac Surg Clin North Am 2016;28(3):409–21.
48. Nicol AL, Hurley RW, Benzon HT. Alternatives to opioids in the pharmacologic management of chronic pain syndromes: a narrative review of randomized, controlled, and blinded clinical trials. Anesth Analg 2017;125(5):1682–703.

Anesthesia and Enhanced Recovery After Head and Neck Surgery

Douglas M. Worrall, MD[a], Anthony Tanella, MD[b],
Samuel DeMaria Jr, MD[b], Brett A. Miles, DDS, MD[a],*

KEYWORDS

- Enhanced recovery • Fast track surgery • Major head and neck surgery
- Preoperative carbohydrate loading • Evidence-based medicine • Surgical outcomes
- Length of stay • Cost

KEY POINTS

- Enhanced recovery after surgery (ERAS) protocols has been shown in a broad range of surgical populations to reduce length of stay and hospital cost with no change in readmission or complication rates.
- Preoperative carbohydrate loading before major surgery has been demonstrated in randomized controlled trials and systematic reviews to increase patient comfort and decrease length of hospitalizations.
- Postoperative aspirin use has not been demonstrated to improve microvascular free flap survival but has been associated with increased risk of hematoma and return to the operating room.
- Multimodal analgesia entails controlling pain by utilizing several classes of analgesic medications to reduce doses and adverse effects of each individual medication.
- The evolution of dedicated specialty-specific intermediate care units has allowed a shift in practices following microvascular head and neck reconstruction to often bypass the intensive care unit with a reduction in length of stay without compromising quality of care.

INTRODUCTION

Enhanced recovery after surgery (ERAS) protocols were pioneered in the late 1990s by colorectal and thoracic surgeons looking for ways to expedite patient recovery.

Disclosure Statement: The authors have nothing to disclose.
[a] Department of Otolaryngology, Head and Neck Surgery, Icahn School of Medicine at Mount Sinai, One Gustave L. Levy Place Box 1189, New York, NY 10029, USA; [b] Department of Anesthesiology, Icahn School of Medicine at Mount Sinai, One Gustave L. Levy Place Box 1010, New York, NY 10029, USA
* Corresponding author.
E-mail address: Brett.Miles@mountsinai.org

Conventional postoperative care after colorectal and thoracic surgery often consisted of a lengthy in-hospital recovery (ie, 5–10 days) with significant postoperative complications.[1–4] To their surprise, surgical technique had limited impact on patient recovery (eg, laparoscopy vs laparotomy). However, reduced length of stay and overall complications could be achieved through standardization of several aspects of patient care during the perioperative period (**Fig. 1**).

The basic tenets of ERAS are that major surgery leads to a significant stress response. The magnitude of this stress correlates with postoperative complications and length of stay, and this can be addressed in several ways[5,6]:

- A multidisciplinary team working together to reduce the impact of surgery
- A multimodal approach to resolving issues that delay recovery and cause complications
- A standardized, evidence-based approach to all phases of perioperative care
- Changes in management using interactive and continuous audits.

Building upon the initial studies in colorectal surgery in Europe, the ERAS Society (http://www.erassociety.org), a nonprofit medical society, was formed in 2010 to promote, develop, and implement ERAS programs. The society publishes guidelines that summarize best practices in patient care for nearly every surgical subspecialty.

SUCCESSFUL IMPLEMENTATION AND INSTITUTIONAL CHANGE

ERAS pathways have been successfully employed in the research setting. However, sustainable adoption in clinical practice requires leveraging organizational change. The authors propose a simple algorithm based on literature surrounding organizational change to promote successful implementation of an ERAS pathway.

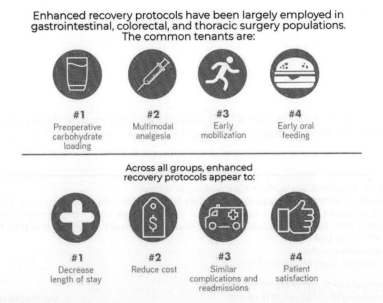

Enhanced recovery protocols have been largely employed in gastrointestinal, colorectal, and thoracic surgery populations. The common tenants are:

#1 Preoperative carbohydrate loading

#2 Multimodal analgesia

#3 Early mobilization

#4 Early oral feeding

Across all groups, enhanced recovery protocols appear to:

#1 Decrease length of stay

#2 Reduce cost

#3 Similar complications and readmissions

#4 Patient satisfaction

Fig. 1. Overview of ERAS protocols.

The first step to bringing about sustainable organizational change is to define the need and couple it to a sense of urgency to fix the problem.[7–11] Successful organizational innovation requires a champion to advocate for change.[10,12,13] Champions should have influence within the organization, the ability to energize the initiative, and skills and power to negotiate with stakeholders.

In the complex multidisciplinary health care environment, a team of champions from different disciplines working toward a shared goal creates a critical mass for successful implementation.[14] Furthermore, change developed by individuals within the institution is far more effective than innovation perceived to be designed by outsiders.[12] Finally, change can be short-lived with premature declaration of victory[15] or when encountering setbacks. Lewin developed a 3-step model to support sustainable change in the face of adversity[9,16,17]:

1. Unfreezing – create dissatisfaction with the status quo, use benchmarks from other organizations, showcase how the benefits of change outweigh the anxiety and negatives associated with change.
2. Moving – implement the innovation with ongoing analysis and subsequent action - an iterative approach to refining the innovation
3. Refreezing – realign organizational norms and culture to support the change and ongoing innovation

By combining these theories of organizational change and the concept of champions, the authors developed a simple algorithm to aid with the adoption of a multidisciplinary ERAS protocol in major head and neck surgery (**Fig. 2**).

ENHANCED RECOVERY AFTER SURGERY FOR MAJOR HEAD AND NECK SURGERY
Preoperative Interventions

Patient education
Conventional presurgical patient education regarding a surgical procedure is limited to the explanation of treatment options during a preoperative clinic visit, the surgical consent process, and/or the preoperative discussion with the anesthesiologist. However, enhanced preoperative patient counseling regarding the anesthetic plan and preoperative and postoperative course, in addition to the surgical procedure, may allay patient anxiety and reduce overall stress.[18,19]

In the context of the bio-behavioral model of stress[18,20] (**Fig. 3**), preoperative patient education reduces patient stress, which may impact wound healing, complications, and even cancer recurrence.[20] Patients undergoing major head and neck cancer surgery are likely to derive the greatest benefits, as their wound healing is complex, requires long-term maintenance care, and is at highest risk of complications.[1–3,21] Managing expectations early and providing information set the stage for a better recovery overall.

Nutrition & reduced fasting guidelines
Many head and neck cancer patients often (18%-57%) suffer from malnutrition caused by mechanical obstruction and tumor cytokines.[22] Malnutrition puts these patients at increased risk of postoperative complications, including refeeding syndrome, poor wound healing, infection, and increased length of stay.

All patients presenting with head and neck cancers should be assessed for malnutrition using a validated nutritional assessment tool.[23] Patients at high risk for malnutrition should be referred to a dietician for counseling. When possible, patients may benefit from delaying surgery to improve nutritional status, which will aid in wound healing (so-called prehabilitation). Currently there are limited

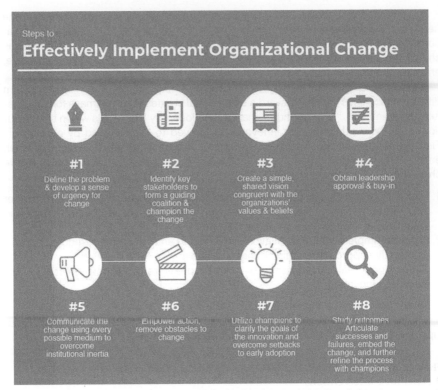

Fig. 2. Proposed methodology to successfully implement organizational change.

data available to determine who would benefit from such a strategy, or to guide decision making for patients preoperatively for prophylactic gastrostomy or a feeding tube.[24]

Conventional beliefs regarding preoperative fasting are nothing by mouth after midnight the day before surgery. Nothing by mouth after midnight may cause dehydration, increase anxiety and physiologic surgical stress, and induce a catabolic state, increasing insulin resistance and perioperative hyperglycemia.[25]

Dehydration will be most prevalent in the later day cases and may lead to hemodynamic instability intraoperatively. Intraoperative and postoperative hyperglycemia from surgical stress and catabolism is associated with increased risk of infection, atrial fibrillation, heart failure, myocardial infarction, pericarditis, neurologic complications, and pulmonary complications.[26,27] In addition, nothing by mouth after midnight may be misinterpreted as forgoing indicated preoperative medications such as beta blockers and aspirin, which reduce the risk of perioperative adverse cardiac events in specific patient populations.[28]

Preoperative fasting guidelines are published by the American Society of Anesthesiologists (ASA) to minimize risk of aspiration during surgery and are more liberal and patient-centric than the traditional nothing by mouth after midnight. The current fasting guidelines (2017) include recommendations for several categories of enteral nutrition as outlined in **Fig. 4**.[29] These guidelines assume normal gastrointestinal anatomy and motility and apply to elective procedures requiring general anesthesia, regional anesthesia, or sedation. Given that many patients undergoing major head and neck surgery

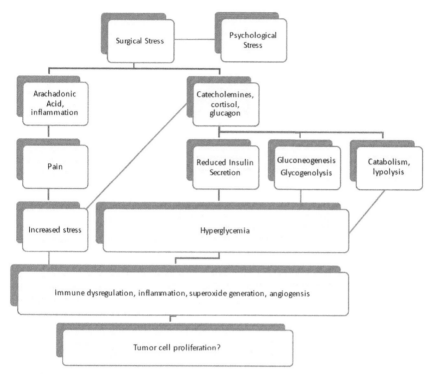

Fig. 3. The surgical stress response and its impact on glucose regulation. (*Data from* Ricon I, Hanalis-Miller T, Haldar R, Jacoby R, Ben-Eliyahu S. Perioperative biobehavioral interventions to prevent cancer recurrence through combined inhibition of beta-adrenergic and - cyclooxygenase 2 signaling. *Cancer.* 2019;125(1):45-56 and Duggan EW, Carlson K, Umpierrez GE. Perioperative Hyperglycemia Management: An Update. *Anesthesiology.* 2017;126(3):547-560.)

have other comorbidities that delay gastric emptying or increase the risk of aspiration (gastroesophageal reflux disease, diabetes mellitus, opioid use and/or altered anatomy along the upper aerodigestive tract), the authors' institution uses the cutoff of 8 hours of fasting for solid foods.

Glucose Loading

In patients not at increased risk of aspiration, consuming carbohydrate-rich clear liquids up to 2 hours prior to their procedure may confer other benefits beyond maintaining normovolemia.[30] Surgical stress induces insulin resistance and hyperglycemia.[25] Hyperglycemia may lead to complications mentioned previously, but particularly concerning are surgical site infections.[26,27,31] Carbohydrate loading reduces preoperative gluconeogenesis, glycogen depletion, and insulin resistance caused by surgical stress (see **Fig. 3**). This in turn will reduce likelihood of perioperative hyperglycemia and associated complications. In addition, it may reduce patient anxiety, thirst, hunger, and malaise, as the less liberal (and dehydrating) liquid intake guidelines are a challenge for most patients.[30] Although it can be assumed that many patients undergoing major surgery for head and neck cancer may be at increased risk for aspiration, the opposite is also true, and many patients are likely to benefit from preoperative carbohydrate loading when appropriate.

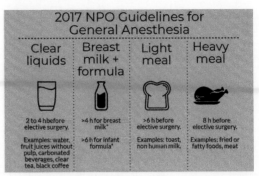

Fig. 4. Updated nil per os (NPO) guidelines for elective surgery. Insufficient evidence exists to evaluate the timing of ingestion of breast milk and infant formula, and current guidelines reflect historic practice. * indicates "Category B1-E evidence". (*Data from* Force ASoAT. Practice Guidelines for Preoperative Fasting and the Use of Pharmacologic Agents to Reduce the Risk of Pulmonary Aspiration: Application to Healthy Patients Undergoing Elective Procedures: An Updated Report *Anesthesiology.* 2017;126(3):376-393.)

Day of surgery presurgical interventions

Preemptive analgesia with oral acetaminophen[32] and gabapentin[33,34] is associated with reduced postoperative pain scores without conferring significant adverse effects. However, the authors recommend caution when administering gabapentin in the elderly (ie, >65 years sold) given altered pharmacokinetics,[35] possible contribution to altered mental status,[36] and the high incidence of postoperative sedation.[33]

Premedication with short-acting benzodiazepine should be considered in especially anxious patients to reduce perioperative stress and catecholamine secretion. Although sedatives may be contraindicated in patients with impending airway collapse, patients presenting for elective head and neck cancer resections may safely receive benzodiazepines to aid in awake bronchoscopic intubations or simply for anxiolysis. Benzodiazepines will have the added benefit of increasing the seizure threshold given the concern of lidocaine toxicity with airway topicalization. Using short-acting agents like midazolam has not been shown to impact the timing or success of postsurgical extubation.[37]

Antibiotic prophylaxis

Antibiotic prophylaxis given within 1 hour of surgery and continued for 24 hours afterward to reduce the rate of surgical site infections (SSIs) is well-established in clean contaminated head and neck oncologic surgery.[38–41] Additionally, antibiotic prophylaxis is given in those for whom the development of an SSI would be disproportionately severe, such as those who would require the removal of an implant or are experiencing free-flap failure.[41–43] Collaboration between multidisciplinary societies[41] recommends cefazolin or cefuroxime plus metronidazole, ampicillin-sulbactam, or clindamycin (in the β lactam allergic patient) for perioperative antibiotic prophylaxis for 24 hours following a clean contaminated head and neck cancer case.

Several studies have shown clindamycin alone to have significantly higher rates of SSIs, fistulas, distant infections, and methicillin-resistant *Staphylococcus aureus* (MRSA) infections, compared with other perioperative antibiotics after controlling for confounders.[43,44] Longer courses of antibiotics have shown no benefit over 24 hours of antibiotics, particularly after controlling for the antibiotic used.[42,43,45–48]

Topical antimicrobial decolonization through the use of chlorhexidine gluconate may reduce the risk of postoperative surgical infections. Topical chlorhexidine oral rinses have been shown to reduce the total oral bacterial colony count by 85%[49] and studies in post-cardiac surgery population have shown a reduction in ventilator associated pneumonia with the addition of chlorhexidine.[50,51] Among head and neck surgery patients, it may be beneficial, as a trend has been shown toward a reduction in SSIs with the addition of perioperative topical antimicrobial decolonization.[52]

Intraoperative Interventions

Normothermia

The rapid redistribution of body heat and reduction in core temperature is the result of anesthetics inhibiting the protective sympathetic peripheral vasoconstriction that occurs in awake patients in cold environments.[53] Hypothermia is associated with poor outcomes, including adverse cardiac events, wound infection, and bleeding.[21,54–57] Intraoperative hypothermia may also affect graft patency, drug pharmacokinetics, and interfere with coagulation.[58] Postemergent hypothermia leads to shivering thermogenesis, which increases metabolic rate and oxygen consumption, increasing risk of flap and vital organ hypoxia. Given the impact of core temperature on morbidity, it is not surprising that intraoperative hypothermia is associated with increased length of stay and cost of care,[59,60] making intraoperative normothermia a key element to any ERAS program.

Hemodynamics, fluid management, and graft function

Under- or over-resuscitating patients has the potential to cause decreased renal perfusion, ileus, coagulopathy, microvascular graft thrombosis, and significant pulmonary or cardiac complications necessitating prolonged hospital stays.[61,62] Goal-directed fluid therapy (GDFT) relies on titrating fluids (either colloid or crystalloid) to hemodynamic variables (eg, pulse pressure variation [PPV], cardiac output/index, or central venous oxygen saturation). Optimum fluid management entails keeping the patient at the peak of the Frank Starling curve, where cardiac output and oxygen delivery are maximized. This optimization of tissue perfusion would logically be beneficial for free tissue transfer survival and wound healing.

Historically, there was concern for vasoconstrictor use affecting flap microcirculation; however, intermittent intraoperative vasoconstrictor use has not been associated with detrimental outcomes during free tissue transfer.[63,64] As a result, graft perfusion is best managed by maintaining normovolemia while minimizing large fluctuations in mean arterial blood pressures with vasoconstricting agents.

Anesthetic plan

The anesthetic plan is broken down into the induction of anesthesia, maintenance, and emergence. The airway management for a head and neck cancer patient can be challenging. Good communication between the surgeon and anesthesia provider to discuss likelihood of intubation success and having an airway plan in place prior to the induction of anesthesia is critical. Routine tracheostomy should be avoided.

When maintaining anesthesia, short-term agents are preferred, as prolonged mechanical ventilation, neuromuscular blockade, or adverse effects from residual agents are seen with long-acting agents.[65,66] Furthermore, limited human data exist showing an association between volatile anesthetics and cancer metastasis.[67] Results of ongoing randomized controlled trials such as General Anesthetics in CAncer REsection Surgery (GA-CARES Trial - NCT03034096) are awaited to evaluate whether general anesthetic choice impacts long-term cancer morbidity and mortality. In light of ongoing work, consider avoiding inhaled anesthetics such as desflurane, sevoflurane, and isoflurane in favor of short-acting intravenous general anesthetics or total intravenous anesthesia (TIVA). Propofol is a short-acting intravenous anesthetic agent capable of inducing and maintaining general anesthesia for a TIVA regimen. With its first-pass hepatic metabolism, it is rapidly cleared and increases the likelihood of extubation at the conclusion of the surgery. Consistent with the tenets of ERAS, multimodal analgesia is initiated the day of surgery. When possible, regional blocks can be performed to aide in postoperative pain control and in some instances improve hemostasis and surgical visualization.[68]

Ventilation strategies

Recommendations for ventilation in ERAS protocols have developed in the thoracic surgery population to avoid postoperative pulmonary complications such as reintubation, pneumonia, and acute respiratory distress syndrome.[69] Lung-protective strategies entail utilizing tidal volumes of 4 to 6 mL/kg of ideal body weight, positive end-expiratory pressure (PEEP) of at least 5 to 10 cm H_2O, limiting peak pressures to less than 30 cm H_2O, frequent recruitment maneuvers, and avoiding overhydration.[69,70] Although data in head and neck surgery are limited, these protective strategies may offer similar benefits in this population.

Postoperative nausea and vomiting prophylaxis

Postoperative nausea and vomiting (PONV) rates for patients receiving anesthesia and surgery are 50%, and 30% without the use of PONV prophylaxis respectively.[71] In light of this and the complexities associated with head and neck free flap surgeries, it is critically important to prevent heaving, retching, and vomiting, as it may compromise a newly reconstructed airway or contribute to graft failure. PONV prophylaxis should be employed in every head and neck cancer case. If a patient is at especially high risk of having PONV, additional precautions should be taken. High risk populations include[71]

1. Women
2. Age younger than 50 years
3. Nonsmoker
4. History of PONV or motion sickness
5. Duration of surgery (longer = higher risk)
6. Patient requiring postoperative opioids
7. Patients receiving general anesthesia
8. Volatile and nitrous oxide exposure

Even in the lowest-risk populations (0 risk factors) there is still a 10% chance of PONV. The rate of PONV increases if risk factors are positive: 20% for one, 40% for two, 60% for three, and 80% for four.[71] To reduce the risk of PONV, inhaled anesthetics are avoided in favor of propofol infusions. Often as part of a standard ENT (ear, nose, and throat) protocol, dexamethasone is administered and has the dual effect of reducing postoperative airway edema and providing PONV prophylaxis at the standard 0.5 to 1 mg/kg dose (max 10 mg). A 5HT3 receptor antagonist, such as ondansetron, should be administered during every case because of a low adverse effect profile and proven efficacy in preventing PONV.

Major head and neck surgery patients are already at high risk for PONV because of the long surgery, postoperative opioids, and general anesthesia and should receive preincision dexamethasone and ondansetron. If any additional risk factors are present, there is an 80% risk of PONV, and additional prophylaxis of up to 3 more antiemetics such as butyrophenones, anticholinergics, and/or Nk-1 receptor antagonists, is recommended.[71] Classes of antiemetics are

- 5-HT3 receptor antagonists (eg, ondansetron)
- Nk-1 receptor antagonists (eg, aprepitant)

- Corticosteroids (eg, dexamethasone)
- Butyrophenones (eg, haloperidol)
- Antihistamines (eg, meclizine)
- Anticholinergics (eg, scopolamine)
- Phenothiazines (eg, metoclopramide)

Postoperative Interventions

Flap monitoring

Given the advances in instrumentation and microvascular technique, the current success rate for free tissue transfer ranges from 90% to 99%.[72–74] However, pedicle thrombosis and subsequent ischemia remain key concerns of the head and neck reconstructive surgeon and warrant prompt detection. Postoperative free flap monitoring instruments and protocols vary between surgeons and institutions. Conventional clinical bedside monitoring of flap color, capillary refill, turgor, temperature, and pinprick testing remains the mainstay of postoperative flap monitoring techniques.[48,75–77] Buried head and neck free flaps require either modification of flap design to allow for an external skin paddle for conventional clinical monitoring or alternative monitoring methods such as a surface or implantable Doppler. Adjunctive measures such as near-infrared spectroscopy, laser Doppler flowmetry, and implantable oxygen partial pressure monitors have undergone experimental testing and may improve flap salvage rate but are often expensive, not widely available, and lack a strong evidence base to support their use compared with clinical monitoring.[76,78]

Prompt detection of ischemia and early re-exploration is ideal. Animal studies showed 100% flap survival after 1 to 4 hours of ischemia, 80% flap survival at 8 hours of ischemia, and 0% flap survival at 12 hours of ischemia.[79] Most free flap compromise occurs within the first 24 hours, and the overwhelming majority of cases occurs within the first 48 hours. Yang and colleagues[80] found 55% of flap compromise occurred within the first 24 hours, 38% from 24 to 48 hours, and 6% after 48 hours. Furthermore, salvage success was also much higher in those flaps noted to be compromised within the first 16 hours (62.2%) compared with those detected after the first 16 hours (21.4%).[80] Therefore, although there has been no randomized trial investigating the frequency or overall duration of free flap monitoring in terms of free flap outcomes, intensive monitoring, every 1 to 4 hours should be maintained during the first 24 to 48 hours postoperatively.[48,77,81,82]

Antiplatelet, anticoagulation management

Mechanical and pharmacologic prophylaxis with subcutaneous low molecular weight heparin or subcutaneous enoxaparin to reduce the risk of venous thromboembolism (VTE) among patients undergoing major head and neck surgery has been well established.[48,83–85] However, anticoagulant use also increases the risk of bleeding complications, particularly in those with concomitant use of antiplatelet medications.[86] No anticoagulant or antithrombotic agent has been shown to improve free flap survival.[48,87–90] Routine aspirin use (without cardiac indication) appears to have no impact on flap failure but significantly increases the risk of postoperative bleeding complications despite its widespread use at many centers performing these procedures.[87,89] Other medications such as dextran, milrinone, and intravenous heparin similarly show no improvement in free flap survival, and are associated with increased complications.[88,89,91,92] As a result, no anticoagulant or antiplatelet agent is routinely recommended to reduce the risk of pedicle thrombosis or flap necrosis.

Pain management

Postoperatively, multimodal analgesia through the use of acetaminophen, local anesthetic wound infiltration, nonsteroidal anti-inflammatory drugs (NSAIDs), gabapentin, and opioids effectively treats pain, facilitates rapid recovery, and minimizes the dose of opioids used and their associated adverse effects (sedation, PONV, pruritis and ileus).[48,93,94] Regional anesthesia may be effective depending on the surgical site, and donor sites should be infiltrated with long-acting local anesthetics.[68] The addition of gabapentin appears to provide excellent perioperative pain relief and reduced postoperative opioid consumption.[95–101]

Ketorolac, celecoxib, and other NSAIDs have been examined in large surgical cohorts and appear to provide effective analgesia without a significant increased risk of bleeding.[102–104] However, among head and neck surgery populations undergoing free flap reconstruction, there appears to be a synergistic increase in bleeding risk when NSAIDs are combined with pharmacologic VTE prophylaxis and/or aspirin.[86,105,106] As a result, the use of NSAIDs in this population should be individualized, and further studies are needed to quantify the bleeding risk to analgesic benefit in this surgical subpopulation. Finally, particularly in those patients with inadequate pain control, patient-controlled analgesia (PCA) has been shown to effectively reduce pain scores.[107,108]

Reflux management

Proton pump inhibitors (PPIs) are often used after major upper aerodigestive tract surgery to reduce the acidity of the reflux, thereby causing less tissue damage and promoting wound healing.[109] In a randomized trial after total laryngectomy, 14 days of a PPI postoperatively significantly reduced the rate of pharyngocutaneous fistula from 32% to 5%.[110] Furthermore, it is postulated that gastroesophageal reflux plays a role in the etiology of head and neck squamous cell carcinoma (HNSCC) and in an epidemiologic study, PPIs and histamine-2 receptor blockers were associated with improved overall survival in HNSCC.[109]

Nicotine replacement therapy

Nicotine replacement therapy is controversial. Although the harms of continuing to smoke tobacco are clear, and surgery represents a unique opportunity to motivate patients to quit, the effect of nicotine replacement therapy (NRT) in the perioperative period is not well-substantiated.[111,112] Nicotine acts as a vasoconstrictor causing tissue hypoxia, flap ischemia, reduced anastomotic patency, impaired bone healing, and failed osseointegration of implants in animal studies.[112–116] Clinically, nicotine replacement has been associated with increased mortality after coronary artery bypass and in patients hospitalized in the medical intensive care unit (ICU).[117,118] Furthermore, there is a dose-dependent increase in wound healing complications in smokers based on their preoperative cotinine levels.[119] Although elective procedures can be delayed until smoking cessation is achieved, major head and neck oncologic surgery should not be delayed to achieve smoking cessation. Given the risk of impaired wound healing and flap ischemia and necrosis, NRT immediately following major head and neck surgery is not currently recommended. Instead these patients should be referred to smoking cessation services preoperatively and may continue postoperatively while further research is done to determine the safety and efficacy of perioperative NRT after major head and neck surgery.

Early mobilization and pulmonary physical therapy

Early and frequent mobilization on postoperative day one (or sooner if possible) is a universal tenet of ERAS protocols across surgical populations.[4,107,120–124] Similarly, within the major head and neck surgery population, early mobilization is critical.[125] Obviously, this can be a challenge with lower extremity donor site morbidity, but the benefits of early mobilization are clear. Furthermore, pulmonary physical therapy in the form incentive spirometry, deep breathing exercises, and intermittent positive pressure breathing reduces postoperative pulmonary complications in other postsurgical populations and should be considered after major head and neck surgery.[48,126]

Early diet initiation

Early oral diet initiation remains an essential and universal component of ERAS programs.[120–122] However, in a major head and neck oncologic population prone to aspiration, wound dehiscence, fistula, and SSIs, there is an understandable hesitancy to initiate an early oral diet. Although gastrointestinal surgeries involving esophagectomy and gastrectomy have shown a decrease length of hospital stay with unchanged or lower complication rates after early oral diet initiation,[122,124,127] the data following major head and neck surgery are sparse.

Traditionally, major head and neck patients have been kept nothing by mouth for 6 to 12 days.[128] However, early oral diet initiation on postoperative day (POD) 1 to 5 after total laryngectomy with primary closure has not been shown to increase pharyngocutaneous fistula rates but also did not reduce hospital length of stay.[129,130] A retrospective review found that free-flap patients fed on or before POD 5 had significantly shorter length of stay (11.9 vs 18 days) and no difference in complications.[128] Currently, major head and neck surgery ERAS programs often give enteral feeding on POD 1 and avoid setting a standardized oral diet initiation day in the protocol. Oral intake is then individualized based on the resection, reconstruction, aspiration risk, and patient characteristics.[48,125] Finally, the adjunctive use of immunonutrition (standard nutritional formulas with the addition amino acids [arginine and glutamine], ribonucleic acid [RNA], and/or lipids), may reduce the risk of fistula formation (11.3% to 5.4%).[131]

Tracheostomy management

Traditionally, after major head and neck surgery with free flap reconstruction, patients would either remain intubated in the ICU or would routinely have a tracheotomy given concerns of oropharyngeal edema and bleeding.[48,125] There has been a shift toward avoidance of routine tracheostomies given the association with increased lower respiratory tract infections, dysphagia, feeding tube dependence, and prolonged hospital stays.[132–134] For those who do require tracheostomy, early cuff deflation, a capping trial, and subsequent decannulation are recommended.[48,125] Finally, surgical closure of the strap muscles and tracheotomy skin incision after decannulation under local anesthesia may decrease length of stay, facilitate swallowing recovery, and have fewer long-term tracheal complications.[135]

Early extubation and routine postoperative intensive care unit admission

Historic trends of routine admission to the ICU of major head and neck surgery patients have largely shifted to intermediate units with specialty trained nursing staff. Postoperative care remains complex. However, the evolution of dedicated high-dependency units (HDUs), specialty trained nonintensive care units at tertiary care centers, has increased availability of high-level, surgery-specific care with similar or improved outcomes and a decreased total cost.[77] Proposed requirements of a dedicated major head and neck HDU are outlined in **Fig. 5**.

Patients kept ventilated and sedated in the ICU after major head and neck surgery with free flap reconstruction have higher rates of pneumonia, more problems weaning

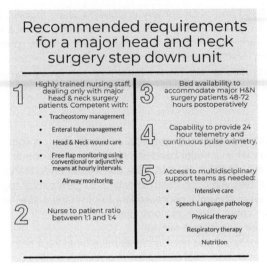

Fig. 5. Proposed requirements of a dedicated major head and neck surgery nonintensive care unit.

from ventilation, and respiratory insufficiency, compared with those allowed to breathe spontaneously and bypass the ICU.[82] Despite the growing utilization of HDUs, there exists a subset of the major head and neck surgery population that will require ICU stay. Varadarajan and colleagues[77] proposed that any of the following could be indications for postoperative ICU admission:

- Patients requiring assisted ventilation
- Patients requiring diagnostic or therapeutic bronchoscopy
- Patients requiring invasive cardiac monitoring such as in the setting of hemodynamic instability
- Patients with multiorgan failure requiring critical care comanagement.

Others are more conservative, recommending that all those deemed at high risk for complications such as those who had bilateral neck dissections, massive blood transfusions, or early return to the operating room to manage a complication, be diverted to the ICU in the immediate postoperative period.[48,136] Overall, there is a trend toward early extubation and immediate postoperative recovery in a specialty unit given the reduction in total cost of care without sacrificing the quality of care. As a result, ICU admissions are reserved for patients with severe medical comorbidities or hemodynamic instability necessitating critical care.

Wound care
Wound care following major head and neck surgery must be tailored to the surgical procedure. Although numerous dressing options exist, split-thickness skin graft donor sites appear to have the most rapid healing and decreased pain and infection risk with hydrocolloid dressings.[137,138] Furthermore, active drains appear superior to passive drains following neck dissection with more rapid healing and adherence of skin flaps and no instances of pedicle compromise due to active drains.[139] Finally, negative pressure or vacuum-assisted closure therapy is safe in major head and neck surgery with free tissue transfer aiding in the healing of complex cervical wounds or over skin graft recipient sites, in which it was shown to ensure better graft acceptance

compared with the traditional bolster technique (81% vs 64% respectively) and decreased total healing times (67 vs 163 days respectively).[140]

SUMMARY

ERAS protocols have been widely developed, substantiated, and practiced in other surgical populations with clear benefits. The application of universal ERAS tenants and evidence based best practices to a major head and neck surgery population offers the opportunity to significantly improve patient outcomes, decrease length of stay, and reduce cost.

REFERENCES

1. Bianchi B, Copelli C, Ferrari S, et al. Free flaps: outcomes and complications in head and neck reconstructions. J Craniomaxillofac Surg 2009;37(8):438–42.
2. Damian D, Esquenazi J, Duvvuri U, et al. Incidence, outcome, and risk factors for postoperative pulmonary complications in head and neck cancer surgery patients with free flap reconstructions. J Clin Anesth 2016;28:12–8.
3. Broome M, Juilland N, Litzistorf Y, et al. Factors influencing the incidence of severe complications in head and neck free flap reconstructions. Plast Reconstr Surg Glob Open 2016;4(10):e1013.
4. Zehr KJ, Dawson PB, Yang SC, et al. Standardized clinical care pathways for major thoracic cases reduce hospital costs. Ann Thorac Surg 1998;66(3):914–9.
5. Ljungqvist O, Scott M, Fearon KC. Enhanced recovery after surgery: a review. JAMA Surg 2017;152(3):292–8.
6. Fearon KC, Ljungqvist O, Von Meyenfeldt M, et al. Enhanced recovery after surgery: a consensus review of clinical care for patients undergoing colonic resection. Clin Nutr 2005;24(3):466–77.
7. Pettigrew AM, Ferlie E, Mckee L. Shaping strategic change: marking change in large organizations: the case of the national health service 1992. London: Sage Pub.
8. Batras D, Duff C, Smith BJ. Organizational change theory: implications for health promotion practice. Health Promot Int 2016;31(1):231–41.
9. Schein E. Organizational culture and leadership. San Francisco (CA): Josey-Bass; 2010.
10. Rogers E. Diffusion of innovations. 5th edition. New York: Free Press; 2003.
11. Burnes B. Kurt Lewin and the planned approach to change: a re-appraisal. J Manag Stud 2004;41:97–1002.
12. Steckler A, Goodman RM. How to institutionalize health promotion programs. Am J Health Promot 1989;3(4):34–43.
13. O'Loughlin J, Renaud L, Richard L, et al. Correlates of the sustainability of community-based heart health promotion interventions. Prev Med 1998; 27(5 Pt 1):702–12.
14. Scalzi CC, Evans LK, Barstow A, et al. Barriers and enablers to changing organizational culture in nursing homes. Nurs Adm Q 2006;30(4):368–72.
15. Kotter JP. Leading change: why transformation efforts fail. Harv Bus Rev 2007; 85:96 (The Tests of a Leader).
16. Lewin K. Frontiers in group dynamics: concept, method and reality in social science; social equilibria social change. Human Relations 1947;1(1):5–41.
17. Lewin K. Resolving social conflicts and field theory in social science. Washington, DC: American Psychological Association; 1997.

18. Kiecolt-Glaser JK, Page GG, Marucha PT, et al. Psychological influences on surgical recovery. Perspectives from psychoneuroimmunology. Am Psychol 1998; 53(11):1209–18.

19. Egbert LD, Battit GE, Welch CE, et al. Reduction of postoperative pain by encouragement and instruction of patients. a study of doctor-patient rapport. N Engl J Med 1964;270:825–7.

20. Ricon I, Hanalis-Miller T, Haldar R, et al. Perioperative biobehavioral interventions to prevent cancer recurrence through combined inhibition of beta-adrenergic and cyclooxygenase 2 signaling. Cancer 2019;125(1):45–56.

21. Clark JR, McCluskey SA, Hall F, et al. Predictors of morbidity following free flap reconstruction for cancer of the head and neck. Head Neck 2007;29(12): 1090–101.

22. Findlay M, Bauer J, Brown T. Evidence-based practice guidelines for the nutritional management of adult patients withhead and neck cancer. Clin Oncol Soc Aust 2016. Available at: https://wiki.cancer.org.au/australiawiki/index.php? oldid=190257. Accessed September 12, 2019.

23. Ferguson M, Capra S, Bauer J, et al. Development of a valid and reliable malnutrition screening tool for adult acute hospital patients. Nutrition 1999;15(6): 458–64.

24. Brown TE, Crombie J, Spurgin AL, et al. Improving guideline sensitivity and specificity for the identification of proactive gastrostomy placement in patients with head and neck cancer. Head Neck 2016;38(Suppl 1):E1163–71.

25. Duggan EW, Carlson K, Umpierrez GE. Perioperative hyperglycemia management: an update. Anesthesiology 2017;126(3):547–60.

26. Fish LH, Weaver TW, Moore AL, et al. Value of postoperative blood glucose in predicting complications and length of stay after coronary artery bypass grafting. Am J Cardiol 2003;92(1):74–6.

27. Hua J, Chen G, Li H, et al. Intensive intraoperative insulin therapy versus conventional insulin therapy during cardiac surgery: a meta-analysis. J Cardiothorac Vasc Anesth 2012;26(5):829–34.

28. Fleisher LA, Fleischmann KE, Auerbach AD, et al. 2014 ACC/AHA guideline on perioperative cardiovascular evaluation and management of patients undergoing noncardiac surgery: executive summary: a report of the American College of Cardiology/American Heart Association Task Force on Practice Guidelines. Circulation 2014;130(24):2215–45.

29. American Society of Anesthesiologists Committee. Practice guidelines for preoperative fasting and the use of pharmacologic agents to reduce the risk of pulmonary aspiration: application to healthy patients undergoing elective procedures: an updated report. Anesthesiology 2017;126(3):376–93.

30. Bilku DK, Dennison AR, Hall TC, et al. Role of preoperative carbohydrate loading: a systematic review. Ann R Coll Surg Engl 2014;96(1):15–22.

31. Wang ZG, Wang Q, Wang WJ, et al. Randomized clinical trial to compare the effects of preoperative oral carbohydrate versus placebo on insulin resistance after colorectal surgery. Br J Surg 2010;97(3):317–27.

32. Watcha MF, Issioui T, Klein KW, et al. Costs and effectiveness of rofecoxib, celecoxib, and acetaminophen for preventing pain after ambulatory otolaryngologic surgery. Anesth Analg 2003;96(4):987–94.

33. Hurley RW, Cohen SP, Williams KA, et al. The analgesic effects of perioperative gabapentin on postoperative pain: a meta-analysis. Reg Anesth Pain Med 2006; 31(3):237–47.

34. Tiippana EM, Hamunen K, Kontinen VK, et al. Do surgical patients benefit from perioperative gabapentin/pregabalin? A systematic review of efficacy and safety. Anesth Analg 2007;104(6):1545–56.
35. Schmader KE, Baron R, Haanpaa ML, et al. Treatment considerations for elderly and frail patients with neuropathic pain. Mayo Clin Proc 2010;85(3 Suppl): S26–32.
36. Fleet JL, Dixon SN, Kuwornu PJ, et al. Gabapentin dose and the 30-day risk of altered mental status in older adults: a retrospective population-based study. PLoS One 2018;13(3):e0193134.
37. Walker KJ, Smith AF. Premedication for anxiety in adult day surgery. Cochrane Database Syst Rev 2009;(4):CD002192.
38. Dor P, Klastersky J. Prophylactic antibiotics in oral, pharyngeal and laryngeal surgery for cancer: (a double-blind study). Laryngoscope 1973;83(12):1992–8.
39. Johnson JT, Myers EN, Thearle PB, et al. Antimicrobial prophylaxis for contaminated head and neck surgery. Laryngoscope 1984;94(1):46–51.
40. Raine CH, Bartzokas CA, Stell PM, et al. Chemoprophylaxis in major head and neck surgery. J R Soc Med 1984;77(12):1006–9.
41. Bratzler DW, Dellinger EP, Olsen KM, et al. Clinical practice guidelines for antimicrobial prophylaxis in surgery. Surg Infect (Larchmt) 2013;14(1):73–156.
42. Busch CJ, Knecht R, Munscher A, et al. Postoperative antibiotic prophylaxis in clean-contaminated head and neck oncologic surgery: a retrospective cohort study. Eur Arch Otorhinolaryngol 2016;273(9):2805–11.
43. Haidar YM, Tripathi PB, Tjoa T, et al. Antibiotic prophylaxis in clean-contaminated head and neck cases with microvascular free flap reconstruction: a systematic review and meta-analysis. Head Neck 2018;40(2):417–27.
44. Pool C, Kass J, Spivack J, et al. Increased surgical site infection rates following clindamycin use in head and neck free tissue transfer. Otolaryngol Head Neck Surg 2016;154(2):272–8.
45. Vila PM, Zenga J, Jackson RS. Antibiotic prophylaxis in clean-contaminated head and neck surgery: a systematic review and meta-analysis. Otolaryngol Head Neck Surg 2017;157(4):580–8.
46. Liu SA, Tung KC, Shiao JY, et al. Preliminary report of associated factors in wound infection after major head and neck neoplasm operations–does the duration of prophylactic antibiotic matter? J Laryngol Otol 2008;122(4):403–8.
47. Carroll WR, Rosenstiel D, Fix JR, et al. Three-dose vs extended-course clindamycin prophylaxis for free-flap reconstruction of the head and neck. Arch Otolaryngol Head Neck Surg 2003;129(7):771–4.
48. Dort JC, Farwell DG, Findlay M, et al. Optimal perioperative care in major head and neck cancer surgery with free flap reconstruction: a consensus review and recommendations from the enhanced recovery after surgery society. JAMA Otolaryngol Head Neck Surg 2017;143(3):292–303.
49. Balbuena L, Stambaugh KI, Ramirez SG, et al. Effects of topical oral antiseptic rinses on bacterial counts of saliva in healthy human subjects. Otolaryngol Head Neck Surg 1998;118(5):625–9.
50. Nicolosi LN, del Carmen Rubio M, Martinez CD, et al. Effect of oral hygiene and 0.12% chlorhexidine gluconate oral rinse in preventing ventilator-associated pneumonia after cardiovascular surgery. Respir Care 2014;59(4):504–9.
51. Klompas M, Speck K, Howell MD, et al. Reappraisal of routine oral care with chlorhexidine gluconate for patients receiving mechanical ventilation: systematic review and meta-analysis. JAMA Intern Med 2014;174(5):751–61.

52. Shuman AG, Shuman EK, Hauff SJ, et al. Preoperative topical antimicrobial decolonization in head and neck surgery. Laryngoscope 2012;122(11):2454–60.
53. Sessler DI. Perioperative heat balance. Anesthesiology 2000;92(2):578–96.
54. Reynolds L, Beckmann J, Kurz A. Perioperative complications of hypothermia. Best Pract Res Clin Anaesthesiol 2008;22(4):645–57.
55. Frank SM, Fleisher LA, Breslow MJ, et al. Perioperative maintenance of normothermia reduces the incidence of morbid cardiac events. A randomized clinical trial. JAMA 1997;277(14):1127–34.
56. Sumer BD, Myers LL, Leach J, et al. Correlation between intraoperative hypothermia and perioperative morbidity in patients with head and neck cancer. Arch Otolaryngol Head Neck Surg 2009;135(7):682–6.
57. Hill JB, Sexton KW, Bartlett EL, et al. The clinical role of intraoperative core temperature in free tissue transfer. Ann Plast Surg 2015;75(6):620–4.
58. Shenkman B, Budnik I, Einav Y, et al. Model of trauma-induced coagulopathy including hemodilution, fibrinolysis, acidosis, and hypothermia: Impact on blood coagulation and platelet function. J Trauma Acute Care Surg 2017;82(2):287–92.
59. Scott AV, Stonemetz JL, Wasey JO, et al. Compliance with Surgical Care Improvement Project for body temperature management (SCIP Inf-10) is associated with improved clinical outcomes. Anesthesiology 2015;123(1):116–25.
60. Kurz A, Sessler DI, Lenhardt R. Perioperative normothermia to reduce the incidence of surgical-wound infection and shorten hospitalization. Study of Wound Infection and Temperature Group. N Engl J Med 1996;334(19):1209–15.
61. Chong MA, Wang Y, Berbenetz NM, et al. Does goal-directed haemodynamic and fluid therapy improve peri-operative outcomes?: a systematic review and meta-analysis. Eur J Anaesthesiol 2018;35(7):469–83.
62. Corcoran T, Rhodes JE, Clarke S, et al. Perioperative fluid management strategies in major surgery: a stratified meta-analysis. Anesth Analg 2012;114(3):640–51.
63. Chen C, Nguyen MD, Bar-Meir E, et al. Effects of vasopressor administration on the outcomes of microsurgical breast reconstruction. Ann Plast Surg 2010;65(1):28–31.
64. Kelly DA, Reynolds M, Crantford C, et al. Impact of intraoperative vasopressor use in free tissue transfer for head, neck, and extremity reconstruction. Ann Plast Surg 2014;72(6):S135–8.
65. Murphy GS, Szokol JW, Marymont JH, et al. Residual neuromuscular blockade and critical respiratory events in the postanesthesia care unit. Anesth Analg 2008;107(1):130–7.
66. Hunter JM. Reversal of residual neuromuscular block: complications associated with perioperative management of muscle relaxation. Br J Anaesth 2017;119(suppl_1):i53–62.
67. Wu ZF, Lee MS, Wong CS, et al. Propofol-based total intravenous anesthesia is associated with better survival than desflurane anesthesia in colon cancer surgery. Anesthesiology 2018;129(5):932–41.
68. Levine AI, Satish G, De Maria S Jr. Anesthesiology and otolaryngology 2014. New York: Springer.
69. Molena D, Mungo B, Stem M, et al. Incidence and risk factors for respiratory complications in patients undergoing esophagectomy for malignancy: a NSQIP analysis. Semin Thorac Cardiovasc Surg 2014;26(4):287–94.
70. Durkin C, Schisler T, Lohser J. Current trends in anesthesia for esophagectomy. Curr Opin Anaesthesiol 2017;30(1):30–5.

71. Gan TJ, Diemunsch P, Habib AS, et al. Consensus guidelines for the management of postoperative nausea and vomiting. Anesth Analg 2014;118(1):85–113.
72. Singh B, Cordeiro PG, Santamaria E, et al. Factors associated with complications in microvascular reconstruction of head and neck defects. Plast Reconstr Surg 1999;103(2):403–11.
73. Khouri RK, Cooley BC, Kunselman AR, et al. A prospective study of microvascular free-flap surgery and outcome. Plast Reconstr Surg 1998;102(3):711–21.
74. Kroll SS, Schusterman MA, Reece GP, et al. Choice of flap and incidence of free flap success. Plast Reconstr Surg 1996;98(3):459–63.
75. Abdel-Galil K, Mitchell D. Postoperative monitoring of microsurgical free tissue transfers for head and neck reconstruction: a systematic review of current techniques–part I. Non-invasive techniques. Br J Oral Maxillofac Surg 2009; 47(5):351–5.
76. Abdel-Galil K, Mitchell D. Postoperative monitoring of microsurgical free-tissue transfers for head and neck reconstruction: a systematic review of current techniques–part II. Invasive techniques. Br J Oral Maxillofac Surg 2009;47(6): 438–42.
77. Varadarajan VV, Arshad H, Dziegielewski PT. Head and neck free flap reconstruction: what is the appropriate post-operative level of care? Oral Oncol 2017;75:61–6.
78. Chae MP, Rozen WM, Whitaker IS, et al. Current evidence for postoperative monitoring of microvascular free flaps: a systematic review. Ann Plast Surg 2015;74(5):621–32.
79. May JW Jr, Chait LA, O'Brien BM, et al. The no-reflow phenomenon in experimental free flaps. Plast Reconstr Surg 1978;61(2):256–67.
80. Yang Q, Ren ZH, Chickooree D, et al. The effect of early detection of anterolateral thigh free flap crisis on the salvage success rate, based on 10 years of experience and 1072 flaps. Int J Oral Maxillofac Surg 2014;43(9):1059–63.
81. Pattani KM, Byrne P, Boahene K, et al. What makes a good flap go bad? A critical analysis of the literature of intraoperative factors related to free flap failure. Laryngoscope 2010;120(4):717–23.
82. Nkenke E, Vairaktaris E, Stelzle F, et al. No reduction in complication rate by stay in the intensive care unit for patients undergoing surgery for head and neck cancer and microvascular reconstruction. Head Neck 2009;31(11):1461–9.
83. Caprini JA, Arcelus JI, Hasty JH, et al. Clinical assessment of venous thromboembolic risk in surgical patients. Semin Thromb Hemost 1991;17(Suppl 3): 304–12.
84. Buesing KL, Mullapudi B, Flowers KA. Deep venous thrombosis and venous thromboembolism prophylaxis. Surg Clin North Am 2015;95(2):285–300.
85. Shuman AG, Hu HM, Pannucci CJ, et al. Stratifying the risk of venous thromboembolism in otolaryngology. Otolaryngol Head Neck Surg 2012;146(5):719–24.
86. Bahl V, Shuman AG, Hu HM, et al. Chemoprophylaxis for venous thromboembolism in otolaryngology. JAMA Otolaryngol Head Neck Surg 2014;140(11): 999–1005.
87. Lee KT, Mun GH. The efficacy of postoperative antithrombotics in free flap surgery: a systematic review and meta-analysis. Plast Reconstr Surg 2015;135(4): 1124–39.
88. Chang EI, Chang EI, Soto-Miranda MA, et al. Comprehensive evaluation of risk factors and management of impending flap loss in 2138 breast free flaps. Ann Plast Surg 2016;77(1):67–71.

89. Lighthall JG, Cain R, Ghanem TA, et al. Effect of postoperative aspirin on outcomes in microvascular free tissue transfer surgery. Otolaryngol Head Neck Surg 2013;148(1):40–6.

90. Barton BM, Riley CA, Fitzpatrick JC, et al. Postoperative anticoagulation after free flap reconstruction for head and neck cancer: a systematic review. Laryngoscope 2018;128(2):412–21.

91. Disa JJ, Polvora VP, Pusic AL, et al. Dextran-related complications in head and neck microsurgery: do the benefits outweigh the risks? A prospective randomized analysis. Plast Reconstr Surg 2003;112(6):1534–9.

92. Jones SJ, Scott DA, Watson R, et al. Milrinone does not improve free flap survival in microvascular surgery. Anaesth Intensive Care 2007;35(5):720–5.

93. Moiniche S, Kehlet H, Dahl JB. A qualitative and quantitative systematic review of preemptive analgesia for postoperative pain relief: the role of timing of analgesia. Anesthesiology 2002;96(3):725–41.

94. Reagan KML, O'Sullivan DM, Gannon R, et al. Decreasing postoperative narcotics in reconstructive pelvic surgery: a randomized controlled trial. Am J Obstet Gynecol 2017;217(3):325.e1-10.

95. Arumugam S, Lau CS, Chamberlain RS. Use of preoperative gabapentin significantly reduces postoperative opioid consumption: a meta-analysis. J Pain Res 2016;9:631–40.

96. Pandey CK, Priye S, Singh S, et al. Preemptive use of gabapentin significantly decreases postoperative pain and rescue analgesic requirements in laparoscopic cholecystectomy. Can J Anaesth 2004;51(4):358–63.

97. Turan A, Karamanlioglu B, Memis D, et al. The analgesic effects of gabapentin after total abdominal hysterectomy. Anesth Analg 2004;98(5):1370–3.

98. Al-Mujadi H, A-Refai AR, Katzarov MG, et al. Preemptive gabapentin reduces postoperative pain and opioid demand following thyroid surgery. Can J Anaesth 2006;53(3):268–73.

99. Quail J, Spence D, Hannon M. Perioperative gabapentin improves patient-centered outcomes after inguinal hernia repair. Mil Med 2017;182(11):e2052–5.

100. Sanders JG, Dawes PJ. Gabapentin for perioperative analgesia in otorhinolaryngology-head and neck surgery: systematic review. Otolaryngol Head Neck Surg 2016;155(6):893–903.

101. Chiu TW, Leung CC, Lau EY, et al. Analgesic effects of preoperative gabapentin after tongue reconstruction with the anterolateral thigh flap. Hong Kong Med J 2012;18(1):30–4.

102. Gobble RM, Hoang HL, Kachniarz B, et al. Ketorolac does not increase perioperative bleeding: a meta-analysis of randomized controlled trials. Plast Reconstr Surg 2014;133(3):741–55.

103. De Oliveira GS Jr, Agarwal D, Benzon HT. Perioperative single dose ketorolac to prevent postoperative pain: a meta-analysis of randomized trials. Anesth Analg 2012;114(2):424–33.

104. Sekiguchi H, Inoue G, Nakazawa T, et al. Loxoprofen sodium and celecoxib for postoperative pain in patients after spinal surgery: a randomized comparative study. J Orthop Sci 2015;20(4):617–23.

105. Forrest JB, Camu F, Greer IA, et al. Ketorolac, diclofenac, and ketoprofen are equally safe for pain relief after major surgery. Br J Anaesth 2002;88(2):227–33.

106. Schleiffarth JR, Bayon R, Chang KE, et al. Ketorolac after free tissue transfer: a comparative effectiveness study. Ann Otol Rhinol Laryngol 2014;123(6):446–9.

107. Wang D, Kong Y, Zhong B, et al. Fast-track surgery improves postoperative recovery in patients with gastric cancer: a randomized comparison with conventional postoperative care. J Gastrointest Surg 2010;14(4):620–7.
108. Jellish WS, Leonetti JP, Sawicki K, et al. Morphine/ondansetron PCA for postoperative pain, nausea, and vomiting after skull base surgery. Otolaryngol Head Neck Surg 2006;135(2):175–81.
109. Papagerakis S, Bellile E, Peterson LA, et al. Proton pump inhibitors and histamine 2 blockers are associated with improved overall survival in patients with head and neck squamous carcinoma. Cancer Prev Res (Phila) 2014;7(12): 1258–69.
110. Stephenson KA, Fagan JJ. Effect of perioperative proton pump inhibitors on the incidence of pharyngocutaneous fistula after total laryngectomy: a prospective randomized controlled trial. Head Neck 2015;37(2):255–9.
111. Nolan MB, Warner DO. Safety and efficacy of nicotine replacement therapy in the perioperative period: a narrative review. Mayo Clin Proc 2015;90(11): 1553–61.
112. Maa J. A second look at nicotine replacement therapy before surgical procedures. Mayo Clin Proc 2015;90(11):1462–4.
113. Ma L, Sham MH, Zheng LW, et al. Influence of low-dose nicotine on bone healing. J Trauma 2011;70(6):E117–21.
114. Berley J, Yamano S, Sukotjo C. The effect of systemic nicotine on osseointegration of titanium implants in the rat femur. J Oral Implantol 2010;36(3):185–93.
115. Ely PB, Kobayashi I A, Campos JH, et al. Nicotine on rat TRAM flap. Acta Cir Bras 2009;24(3):216–20.
116. Sachar K, Goel R, Weiss AP. Acute and chronic effects of nicotine on anastomotic patency following ischemia/reperfusion. J Reconstr Microsurg 1998; 14(3):179–84.
117. Paciullo CA, Short MR, Steinke DT, et al. Impact of nicotine replacement therapy on postoperative mortality following coronary artery bypass graft surgery. Ann Pharmacother 2009;43(7):1197–202.
118. Lee AH, Afessa B. The association of nicotine replacement therapy with mortality in a medical intensive care unit. Crit Care Med 2007;35(6):1517–21.
119. Rinker B. The evils of nicotine: an evidence-based guide to smoking and plastic surgery. Ann Plast Surg 2013;70(5):599–605.
120. Gemmill EH, Humes DJ, Catton JA. Systematic review of enhanced recovery after gastro-oesophageal cancer surgery. Ann R Coll Surg Engl 2015;97(3):173–9.
121. Feng F, Ji G, Li JP, et al. Fast-track surgery could improve postoperative recovery in radical total gastrectomy patients. World J Gastroenterol 2013;19(23): 3642–8.
122. So JB, Lim ZL, Lin HA, et al. Reduction of hospital stay and cost after the implementation of a clinical pathway for radical gastrectomy for gastric cancer. Gastric Cancer 2008;11(2):81–5.
123. Blom RL, van Heijl M, Bemelman WA, et al. Initial experiences of an enhanced recovery protocol in esophageal surgery. World J Surg 2013;37(10):2372–8.
124. Lee L, Li C, Robert N, et al. Economic impact of an enhanced recovery pathway for oesophagectomy. Br J Surg 2013;100(10):1326–34.
125. Coyle MJ, Main B, Hughes C, et al. Enhanced recovery after surgery (ERAS) for head and neck oncology patients. Clin Otolaryngol 2016;41(2):118–26.
126. Thomas JA, McIntosh JM. Are incentive spirometry, intermittent positive pressure breathing, and deep breathing exercises effective in the prevention of

postoperative pulmonary complications after upper abdominal surgery? A systematic overview and meta-analysis. Phys Ther 1994;74(1):3–10 [discussion: 10–6].

127. Lewis SJ, Egger M, Sylvester PA, et al. Early enteral feeding versus "nil by mouth" after gastrointestinal surgery: systematic review and meta-analysis of controlled trials. BMJ 2001;323(7316):773–6.

128. Guidera AK, Kelly BN, Rigby P, et al. Early oral intake after reconstruction with a free flap for cancer of the oral cavity. Br J Oral Maxillofac Surg 2013;51(3): 224–7.

129. Aires FT, Dedivitis RA, Petrarolha SM, et al. Early oral feeding after total laryngectomy: a systematic review. Head Neck 2015;37(10):1532–5.

130. Seven H, Calis AB, Turgut S. A randomized controlled trial of early oral feeding in laryngectomized patients. Laryngoscope 2003;113(6):1076–9.

131. Howes N, Atkinson C, Thomas S, et al. Immunonutrition for patients undergoing surgery for head and neck cancer. Cochrane Database Syst Rev 2018;(8):CD010954.

132. Coyle MJ, Tyrrell R, Godden A, et al. Replacing tracheostomy with overnight intubation to manage the airway in head and neck oncology patients: towards an improved recovery. Br J Oral Maxillofac Surg 2013;51(6):493–6.

133. Castling B, Telfer M, Avery BS. Complications of tracheostomy in major head and neck cancer surgery; a retrospective study of 60 consecutive cases. Br J Oral Maxillofac Surg 1994;32(1):3–5.

134. Moore MG, Bhrany AD, Francis DO, et al. Use of nasotracheal intubation in patients receiving oral cavity free flap reconstruction. Head Neck 2010;32(8): 1056–61.

135. Brookes JT, Seikaly H, Diamond C, et al. Prospective randomized trial comparing the effect of early suturing of tracheostomy sites on postoperative patient swallowing and rehabilitation. J Otolaryngol 2006;35(2):77–82.

136. de Melo GM, Ribeiro KC, Kowalski LP, et al. Risk factors for postoperative complications in oral cancer and their prognostic implications. Arch Otolaryngol Head Neck Surg 2001;127(7):828–33.

137. Beam JW. Management of superficial to partial-thickness wounds. J Athl Train 2007;42(3):422–4.

138. Sinha S, Schreiner AJ, Biernaskie J, et al. Treating pain on skin graft donor sites: review and clinical recommendations. J Trauma Acute Care Surg 2017;83(5): 954–64.

139. Batstone MD, Lowe D, Shaw RJ, et al. Passive versus active drainage following neck dissection: a non-randomised prospective study. Eur Arch Otorhinolaryngol 2009;266(1):121–4.

140. Bach CA, Guillere L, Yildiz S, et al. Comparison of negative pressure wound therapy and conventional dressing methods for fibula free flap donor site management in patients with head and neck cancer. Head Neck 2016;38(5):696–9.

The Difficult Airway

Carlos A. Artime, MD[a],*, Soham Roy, MD[b], Carin A. Hagberg, MD[c]

KEYWORDS

- Airway management ● Difficult Airway ● Airway obstruction ● Difficult intubation
- Head and neck pathology

KEY POINTS

- The difficult airway in otolaryngologic surgery requires careful planning and close communication between the anesthesiologist and ENT or head and neck surgeon.
- Knowledge of predictive factors and a detailed preoperative evaluation can be used to predict which airway strategies are likely to be successful and which are likely to fail.
- A comprehensive plan should include alternative strategies depending on the occurrence and timing of failure or complications.

INTRODUCTION

Airway management is a cornerstone of anesthetic practice, and difficulty with airway management has potentially grave implications—failure to secure a patent airway can result in hypoxic brain injury or death in a matter of minutes. The *Practice Guidelines for Management of the Difficult Airway* of the American Society of Anesthesiologists (ASA) defines the difficult airway as "the clinical situation in which a conventionally trained anesthesiologist experiences difficulty with ventilation of the upper airway via a mask, difficulty with tracheal intubation, or both."[1] Difficulty with supraglottic airway (SGA) placement and difficulty with surgical airway (front of neck access) are additional considerations.

Because of head and neck pathology and other factors, the incidence of difficult airway is higher in patients undergoing otolaryngologic surgery.[2,3] Common causes for difficulty with airway management in otolaryngologic surgery include, but are not limited to, subglottic stenosis, glottic and supraglottic neoplasm, infection (eg,

Disclosures: None.

[a] Department of Anesthesiology, McGovern Medical School at the University of Texas Health Science Center at Houston, Memorial Hermann Hospital - Texas Medical Center, 6431 Fannin St., MSB 5.020, Houston, TX 77030, USA; [b] Department of Otorhinolaryngology–Head and Neck Surgery, McGovern Medical School at the University of Texas Health Science Center at Houston, Children's Memorial Hermann Hospital, 6431 Fannin St., MSB 5.020, Houston, TX 77030, USA; [c] Anesthesiology, Critical Care & Pain Medicine, Department of Anesthesiology & Perioperative Medicine, University of Texas MD Anderson Cancer Center, 1400 Holcombe Blvd., Unit 409, Houston, TX 77030, USA
* Corresponding author.
E-mail address: carlos.artime@uth.tmc.edu

Ludwig's angina or epiglottitis), prior otolaryngologic surgery, history of radiation to the head and neck, thyromegaly, airway trauma, vocal cord dysfunction, and obstructive sleep apnea.

In 2011, the Royal College of Anaesthetists and the Difficult Airway Society (DAS) of the United Kingdom reported the results of the fourth National Audit Project (NAP4), a 1-year audit that aimed to determine the incidence of major complications of airway management in anesthesia.[4] Out of 133 major airway-related events in the perioperative period, 57 (43%) were associated with head and neck pathology; of these, all but 2 patients were undergoing otolaryngologic surgery. Of the 58 surgical cases in NAP4 where an emergency surgical airway was attempted for a "cannot intubate, cannot oxygenate" (CICO) scenario, 43 (74%) were on the head and neck. Arné and colleagues[3] reported a 12.3% difficult intubation rate in patients with head and neck cancer, compared with 3.5% of those undergoing non-cancer otolaryngologic surgery and 2% of general surgical patients.

PREDICTION OF THE DIFFICULT AIRWAY

A detailed preoperative assessment can identify patient characteristics that are associated with a difficult airway and assist with planning of the airway management strategy. Certain physical findings or details from the patient's history can be prognostic of difficulty with mask ventilation, SGA placement, direct laryngoscopy (DL), video laryngoscopy, or the performance of a surgical airway—many of these are commonly found in patients presenting for otolaryngologic surgery (**Table 1**).

Whenever possible, previous anesthetic records should be examined, especially those involving airway management[1]; one of the most predictive factors for difficult intubation is a history of previous difficulty with intubation.[5] The anesthesiologist should review the ENT surgeon's notes in detail, with specific attention to characterizations of the patient's airway, as well as any results of nasopharyngeal laryngoscopy performed beforehand. Computed tomography of the airway, if performed, should also be examined before formalizing an airway management plan.[6]

A patient history should be elicited, including a review of symptoms that may indicate airway obstruction, such as stridor or paroxysmal nocturnal dyspnea.[7] The preoperative interview should also address the possibility of events having occurred since the last anesthetic such as weight gain; laryngeal stenosis from previous airway intervention, including history of previous tracheostomy; or radiation to the head and neck. The quality of the patient's voice should be noted—a muffled voice may indicate supraglottic pathology, whereas laryngeal lesions result in a coarse, breathy, hoarse, or scratchy voice.[2]

A physical examination should include a visual examination of the face and neck, with special attention for obvious facial deformities, neoplasms involving the face or neck, facial burns, a large goiter, a short or thick neck, or a receding mandible.[8] Assessment of mouth opening, oropharyngeal anatomy, dentition, and mandibular protrusion should be performed. The submandibular space should also be palpated; a finding of small submandibular space (retrognathia) or poor submandibular compliance (due to masses, infection, or radiation changes) is a nonreassuring finding.

Although the ENT surgeon has often already performed a nasopharyngeal laryngoscopy before a planned surgical intervention on the airway, a preoperative endoscopic airway examination (PEAE) performed by the anesthesiologist can assess for any changes since the last office visit and guide airway management planning. In a prospective study by Rosenblatt and colleagues,[9] PEAE influenced the planned airway management strategy in 26% of patients presenting for airway surgery and reduced the need for awake intubation.

Table 1
Clinical predictors of difficulty with different phases of airway management

Difficult Mask Ventilation	• Obstructive sleep apnea or history of snoring • Age older than 55 y • Male gender • Obesity (BMI >30 kg/m²) • Mallampati classification III or IV • Presence of a beard • Edentulousness
Difficult SGA Ventilation	• Male gender • Obesity (BMI >30 kg/m²) • Poor dentition • Neck radiation • Reduced mouth opening • Reduced cervical spine mobility • Tonsillar hypertrophy • Glottic, hypopharyngeal, or subglottic pathology
Difficult Direct Laryngoscopy	• Long upper incisors • Prominent overbite • Inability to protrude mandible • Small mouth opening • Mallampati classification III or IV • High, arched palate • Short thyromental distance • Short, thick neck • Limited cervical mobility
Difficult Video-Assisted Laryngoscopy	• Otolaryngologic and cardiac surgery • Head in the "sniffing" position • Abnormal neck anatomy (scar, mass, radiation changes) • Decreased cervical spine motion • Reduced cervical spine mobility • Restricted oropharyngeal space

Abbreviation: BMI, body mass index.
  Data from Artime C, Hagberg C. Airway Management. In: Miller RD, ed. *Miller's Anesthesia*. 8th ed. Philadelphia, PA: Elsevier 2014, Rosenblatt W, Artime C. Management of the difficult airway for general anesthesia. In: Crowley M, ed. *UpToDate*. UpToDate.com 2019, and Nekhendzy V. Anesthesia for head and neck surgery. In: Crowley M, ed. *UpToDate*. UpToDate.com 2019.

MANAGEMENT OF THE DIFFICULT AIRWAY

When the preoperative evaluation indicates a known or predicted difficult airway in a patient undergoing otolaryngologic surgery, a discussion between the anesthesiologist and ENT surgeon regarding the patient's airway and surgery-specific issues is necessary to devise a detailed airway management strategy. This strategy should include a predetermined set of sequential plans designed to manage failure of previous attempts at airway management and ultimately achieve oxygenation, ventilation, and protection against aspiration.[10] Regardless of the primary airway management strategy, alternative strategies in the event of failure or complications must be preemptively delineated. Different plans may need to be made depending on the type and timing of a complication or at what stage a failure of strategy occurs.[11]

The ASA's *Practice Guidelines for Management of the Difficult Airway* includes a Difficult Airway Algorithm (DAA) intended to guide clinical decision-making when an anesthesiologist is faced with a known or potential difficult airway.[1] This algorithm does not follow a linear decision-making tree, as the ACLS algorithms do. It can be better understood and remembered by considering it as 3 separate scenarios: (1) predicted difficult airway (awake intubation), (2) difficult intubation with adequate oxygenation/ventilation (the "nonemergency" pathway), and (3) difficult intubation without adequate oxygenation/ventilation (the CICO scenario or the "emergency" pathway).[8]

The ASA DAA begins with a consideration of the relative merits and feasibility of 4 basic management choices:

1. Awake intubation versus intubation after induction of general anesthesia,
2. Preservation versus ablation of spontaneous ventilation,
3. Video-assisted laryngoscopy (VAL) as an initial approach to intubation, and
4. Noninvasive techniques versus invasive techniques (ie, surgical or percutaneous airway) for the initial approach to intubation.

Awake Airway Management

The safest plan for a patient who requires endotracheal intubation and has a difficult airway is for that patient to undergo intubation before induction of general anesthesia. Awake intubation should be considered when difficulty with tracheal intubation is anticipated and either: mask ventilation and SGA ventilation are both anticipated to be difficult; the patient will not tolerate an apneic period; or the patient is at high risk for aspiration of gastric contents.[12] Awake intubation is most commonly performed using a flexible intubation scope (FIS),[13] although other techniques have been successfully used, including VAL.[14] The benefits of awake airway management include the preservation of pharyngeal muscle tone and patency of the upper airway, the maintenance of spontaneous ventilation, and a safeguard against aspiration due to the preservation of protective airway reflexes. There are no absolute contraindications to awake intubation other than patient's refusal or a patient who is unable to cooperate (such as a child, an intellectually disabled patient, or a patient with altered mental status).[13]

Extreme caution should be taken in the patient with critical airway obstruction. Even the process of topicalization with local anesthetic can precipitate loss of the airway, as can some of the complications associated with awake intubation (eg, airway bleeding and laryngospasm).[7] These patients require excellent coordination between the anesthesiologist and ENT surgeon; the feasibility and appropriateness of an awake surgical airway should be considered (see later discussion).

Topicalization of the airway with local anesthetics should, in most cases, be the primary anesthetic for awake intubation; many times, it is all that is needed.[13] Topicalization should primarily be focused on the base of the tongue (pressure receptors here act as the afferent component of the gag reflex), the oropharynx, the hypopharynx, and the laryngeal structures; anesthesia of the oral cavity is unnecessary. If a nasotracheal intubation is planned, then the nasal cavity should also be topicalized. Before airway topicalization, an anticholinergic should be administered to aid in the drying of secretions, which helps improve both the effectiveness of the topical local anesthetics and visualization during laryngoscopy.[8]

Depending on the clinical circumstance, intravenous (IV) sedation may be useful in allowing the patient to tolerate awake intubation by providing anxiolysis, amnesia, and analgesia. Benzodiazepines, opioids, hypnotics, alpha-2 agonists, and neuroleptics can be used alone or in combination.[15] It is important that these agents be carefully titrated to effect, as oversedation can render a patient uncooperative and make awake intubation more difficult or result in a lost airway.[13] Careful coordination with the otolaryngologist is essential before any delivery of sedation, as loss of airway in this pathway may necessitate emergent surgical intervention. Spontaneous respiration with adequate oxygenation and ventilation should always be maintained.[15] In patients with critical airway obstruction, sedation should be used sparingly or avoided altogether, as awake muscle tone is sometimes necessary in these patients to maintain airway patency.[16] Avoidance of oversedation is also important in the patient with a full stomach, as an awake patient can protect his or her own airway in the event of regurgitation.[13]

Induction of Anesthesia

Securing the airway after induction of general anesthesia is reasonable if either mask ventilation, SGA ventilation, or endotracheal intubation is likely to be successful. The strategy for induction should consider which aspect of airway management is predicted to be difficult and provide the ability to ensure adequate ventilation and the ability to awaken the patient if necessary. IV induction for endotracheal intubation usually leads to ablation of spontaneous ventilation, although spontaneous ventilation may be preserved using total IV anesthesia as part of a combined surgical and anesthetic plan. An inhalational technique can also be used if the preservation of spontaneous ventilation is preferred.

For IV induction, an adequate dose of short-acting induction agent (usually propofol) should be administered. Too high a dose may delay the return of spontaneous ventilation if necessary for rescue, whereas underdosing may lead to difficulty with mask ventilation or SGA placement. If an opioid is used as part of the induction regimen, a short-acting agent is preferred, and naloxone should be immediately available for reversal should reestablishment of spontaneous ventilation be required.

Neuromuscular blocking drugs (NMBDs) improve intubating conditions by facilitating laryngoscopy and preventing reflexive laryngeal closure and have been demonstrated to improve mask ventilation, especially when difficulty is the result of laryngospasm, opioid-induced rigidity, or light anesthesia. Succinylcholine has the benefit of a rapid onset combined with a short duration of action that theoretically allows for the resumption of spontaneous ventilation before severe hypoxia develops in a preoxygenated patient. Rocuronium is a nondepolarizing NMBD that can be reversed by sugammadex (a selective binding agent) in a time comparable to spontaneous recovery from succinylcholine.

The choice and timing of NMBD administration should depend on the aspect of airway management that is expected to be difficult. Regardless, when IV induction is used for the difficult airway, NMBDs should not be withheld, as this could create a scenario in which mask ventilation and intubation are impossible, or delayed, which could lead to the onset of hypoxia before spontaneous recovery (with succinylcholine) or reversal (with sugammadex) would have been possible. For patients in whom difficulty with both ventilation and intubation is predicted, awake airway management should be performed, and the administration of NMBDs should be avoided until the ability to ventilate is proved.[8]

Inhalation induction can be used when the preservation of spontaneous ventilation is desired and is often chosen for induction of the difficult airway. The concentration of volatile anesthetic (usually sevoflurane) is slowly increased leading to central nervous system depression, usually with the preservation of spontaneous ventilation. Positive pressure ventilation is gradually applied; once ventilation is completely controlled, NMBDs may be administered. If airway obstruction occurs at any point during the induction, the volatile agent can be discontinued, and redistribution results in awakening, typically with resolution of the obstruction.[17]

Inhalation induction has been shown to be effective for management of the difficult airway in otolaryngologic surgery, but may certainly fail and rescue plans must be in place.[4,18] It is of limited value when dealing with a collapsible lesion and should not be performed when mask ventilation is predicted to be difficult.[2,18]

Intubation Techniques Including Video-Assisted Laryngoscopy

DL is the most common technique for endotracheal intubation. However, in the patient with head and neck pathology, particularly glottic or supraglottic tumors, multiple DL attempts can lead to bleeding, edema, and worsening of the ability to ventilate. VAL has been shown to result in improved glottic visualization, compared with DL, in both routine airway management and in the predicted difficult airway, but not those with head and neck lesions or those patients' status postradiation therapy.[1,19] Although this improved visualization does not necessarily translate into increased success with intubation (particularly in the normal airway), studies have demonstrated improved intubation success with VAL in patients with predicted difficult airways.[20,21] Various different videolaryngoscopes have been introduced, each with its own design and specific features. Generally, videolaryngoscopes can be divided into 3 groups: (1) those whose design is based on the Macintosh direct laryngoscope, (2) those that incorporate highly curved or distally angulated blades, and (3) those that incorporate an endotracheal tube (ETT)-guiding channel.[22] Experts recommend a consideration of VAL over DL for the patient with head and neck pathology and a limitation of multiple attempts if DL is chosen as the primary strategy.[2]

The FIS is also extremely useful for management of the difficult airway. It is the most commonly used device for awake intubation and is particularly useful for patients with limited mouth opening or to facilitate nasotracheal intubation. It may have limited utility in certain scenarios because airway bleeding can obscure anatomic landmarks and soil the tip of the FIS with blood, making visualization of the larynx extremely difficult, but bleeding also compromises the utility of VAL as well. Obstruction due to neoplasm or severe airway stenosis may result in the inability to pass the FIS; suspected pathology in these patients should be discussed with the surgical team before instrumentation of the airway, as a surgical airway may be required. Intubation with an FIS can be performed in the awake or anesthetized patient. The major technical disadvantage to using it under general anesthesia is the loss of pharyngeal muscle tone, which can lead to upper airway collapse and resultant difficulty in visualizing the glottis.[23] Therefore, the need to open the airway with either chin lift, jaw thrust, or an oral airway will in most cases be necessary.

Several other devices have a role in management of the difficult airway in otolaryngologic surgery. Rigid optical stylets may be useful in bypassing mobile supraglottic and glottic masses in situations where an FIS is unable to displace the obstructing tissue.[2] The rigid bronchoscope can be used by the ENT surgeon to establish and maintain the airway in patients presenting with obstructing masses, external tracheal compression, and hemorrhage. In contrast to the FIS, the rigid bronchoscope has a ventilation port that can be directly connected to the anesthesia ventilator, allowing for external ventilation while airway procedures are performed.[22] Operative laryngoscopy by the ENT surgeon using the anterior commissure scope has also shown utility in securing a difficult airway when other techniques have failed.[24]

Surgical Airway as a Primary Approach to Airway Management

In patients with critical upper airway obstruction or severe subglottic stenosis, a surgical airway before induction of general anesthesia is potentially the safest option. Awake tracheostomy is most often performed, although awake needle cricothyrotomy has been described as well.[18,25] The most common indication for awake tracheostomy in several case series was upper airway malignancy; most of these patients presented with significant upper airway obstruction and dyspnea.[26,27] Other indications included facial or airway trauma, bilateral vocal cord paralysis, infection, bleeding/hematoma, and glottic or subglottic stenosis.[26,27]

Complications of tracheostomy include displacement of the tracheostomy tube, traumatic injury, and pneumothorax; a higher incidence of complications has not been consistently demonstrated in awake tracheostomy versus after induction of general anesthesia.[27–29] The risks and benefits of proceeding with awake tracheostomy as a primary airway plan must be carefully considered and should be a joint decision between the ENT surgeon and anesthesiologist, accounting for the patient's respiratory status, imaging, and the results of a PEAE.

EXTUBATION OF THE DIFFICULT AIRWAY

A critical component of airway management is the process of extubation. Although significant emphasis is placed on complications that can arise during induction and intubation, the risk can potentially be higher during extubation.[30] In the NAP4 study, one-third of major complications of airway management occurred at extubation or in the recovery room with a mortality rate of 5%; airway obstruction was the most common cause.[4] Analysis of the ASA Closed Claims database has shown that although the number of claims for death and brain damage during intubation has decreased since the initial adoption of the ASA Practice Guidelines, the number of claims arising from injury at extubation and during recovery has remained steady.[31] Specifically, patients recovering from otolaryngologic surgery have been shown to be at higher risk for extubation complications.[32,33]

This is an especially important consideration given the emphasis on early weaning and extubation in most Enhanced Recovery after Surgery protocols for head and neck cancer surgery. Successful extubation depends on 2 factors: the ability to maintain a patent airway once the ETT is removed and the ability to tolerate spontaneous ventilation without mechanical ventilatory support. *Extubation failure* refers to failure of the former, whereas *weaning* or *liberation failure* refers to inability of the latter. Although it is important to ensure that the otolaryngologic surgical patient is able to ventilate without mechanical support, the primary consideration in most cases is whether the patient can maintain a patent airway.[32,34]

When formulating an extubation plan, it is important to stratify not only the risk of extubation failure but also the feasibility of reintubation. Extubation of the difficult airway, therefore, requires special consideration. Although the ASA Practice Guidelines provide some general considerations for extubation of the difficult airway, the DAS produced the first comprehensive guidelines for management of tracheal extubation in adult perioperative practice in 2012 that is invaluable for managing extubation of the difficult airway in otolaryngologic surgery.[35]

Per the DAS guidelines, risk stratification can be accomplished by considering the following: (1) whether the airway was normal and uncomplicated at induction; (2) whether the airway has become difficult to manage as a result of surgical changes, trauma, or nonsurgical factors; and (3) whether the patient has general risk factors for an unsuccessful extubation.[35]

Many surgical and anesthetic factors can increase extubation risk. A summary of the most pertinent factors is listed in **Table 2**. Clearly, if difficulty with mask ventilation or endotracheal intubation was encountered at induction, particular caution should be exercised at the time of extubation due to the expected difficulty of reintubation, if

Table 2	
Factors associated with increased extubation risk	
Airway Risk Factors	• Known difficult airway • Airway deterioration (surgical changes, bleeding, edema, trauma) • Obesity and obstructive sleep apnea • Restricted airway access • Aspiration risk
General Risk Factors	• Cardiovascular disease • Respiratory disease • Neuromuscular disease • Metabolic derangements

Data from Popat M, Mitchell V, Dravid R, et al: Difficult Airway Society Guidelines for the management of tracheal extubation, Anaesthesia 67:318-340, 2012.

needed. Often, there is a higher rate of failed extubation in this scenario due to airway edema as a result of multiple attempts at initially securing the airway. On the other hand, airway management will not be easy after completion of surgery simply because it was easy initially. Thyroidectomy, microlaryngeal surgery, and maxillofacial surgery are only a few examples of otolaryngologic surgical procedures that can lead to a difficult airway at extubation. Many extubation problems associated with surgical procedures involve postoperative bleeding, nerve damage, or direct tissue trauma. Caution should be observed with devices placed near the airway intra- and postoperatively, (eg, maxillomandibular fixation or large dressings on the head or neck). These devices may restrict airway access and lead to difficulty with reintubation.[36]

Communication between the ENT surgeon and anesthesiologist is essential when making the decision on whether or not to extubate a difficult airway. There should be a clear discussion of the risks and benefits of extubation versus prolonged intubation considering the initial airway management, the surgical procedure, and the anticipated recovery timeline. The patient's future operative schedule should be taken into account; it is illogical to extubate a patient with a difficult airway who will be returning for follow-up surgery within a short time period.[36]

Extubation Strategies

Once the decision to extubate has been confirmed, strategies for a safe extubation can be formulated. The anesthesiologist and ENT surgeon should review the various options for extubation and formulate a plan of action to regain control of the airway if extubation fails.

Of the several techniques that can be used to manage extubation of the difficult airway, the use of an airway exchange catheter (AEC) is routine and is recommended by both the DAS and ASA guidelines. AECs are hollow reintubation guides that are passed through an ETT before extubation and kept in place until the potential need for reintubation has passed. They have the additional capability of maintaining oxygenation or monitoring ventilation by attachment to a capnograph. Smaller AECs (11 Fr) are generally well tolerated by awake patients, who can breathe, talk, and cough around them. They should be secured with tape in place to prevent accidental dislodgement and labeled to distinguish them from traditional feeding tubes, which can have a similar appearance. Reintubation over an AEC, if necessary, can be facilitated by DL or VAL to retract the tongue and oropharyngeal soft tissue.[36]

The ASA Practice Guidelines recommend consideration of the risks and benefits of an awake extubation versus extubation in the deeply anesthetized state. Deep extubation has been described in patients with both straightforward and difficult airways and may decrease the risk of coughing and "bucking" before extubation. There is, however, a significant risk of airway obstruction due to the effects of deep anesthesia on pharyngeal muscle tone. Therefore, the investigators feel that this practice should generally be discouraged in the face of a difficult airway and that awake extubation is usually the most appropriate strategy. One exception, however, is the laryngeal mask airway (LMA)-assisted extubation, as described in the DAS guidelines. This technique may play a role in facilitating deep extubation in patients at high risk for extubation failure by acting as a "bridge" to successful extubation. Hemodynamic stress and coughing or bucking have been shown to be reduced during emergence with an LMA in place compared with tracheal extubation in both the awake and deeply anesthetized state.[37,38] A common technique of ETT/LMA exchange is to first place the LMA behind the ETT, a procedure termed the *Bailey maneuver*.[39] Flexible bronchoscopy can be used in combination with an LMA-assisted extubation when evaluation of vocal cord function is an important part of the extubation plan, such as after complex thyroid surgery.[40]

SUMMARY

The difficult airway in otolaryngologic surgery requires careful planning and close communication between the anesthesiologist and ENT or head and neck surgeon. Knowledge of predictive factors and a detailed preoperative evaluation can be used to predict which airway strategies are likely to be successful and which are likely to fail. A comprehensive plan should include alternative strategies depending on the occurrence and timing of failure or complications. The risks associated with the difficult airway extend into the time of extubation and recovery, and a structured approach to extubation is of the utmost importance.

REFERENCES

1. Apfelbaum JL, Hagberg CA, Caplan RA, et al. Practice guidelines for management of the difficult airway: an updated report by the American Society of Anesthesiologists Task Force on Management of the Difficult Airway. Anesthesiology 2013;118(2):251–70.
2. Nekhendzy V, Biro P. Airway management in head and neck surgery. In: Hagberg CA, Artime C, Aziz M, editors. Hagberg and Benumof's airway management. 3rd edition. Philadelphia: Elsevier; 2018. p. 668–91.
3. Arné J, Descoins P, Fusciardi J, et al. Preoperative assessment for difficult intubation in general and ENT surgery: predictive value of a clinical multivariate risk index. Br J Anaesth 1998;80(2):140–6.
4. Cook TM, Woodall N, Frerk C, Fourth National Audit Project. Major complications of airway management in the UK: results of the Fourth National Audit Project of the Royal College of Anaesthetists and the Difficult Airway Society. Part 1: anaesthesia. Br J Anaesth 2011;106(5):617–31.
5. Lundstrom LH, Moller AM, Rosenstock C, et al. A documented previous difficult tracheal intubation as a prognostic test for a subsequent difficult tracheal intubation in adults. Anaesthesia 2009;64(10):1081–8.
6. Artime CA, Hagberg CA. Awake Intubation. In: Abdelmalak B, Doyle DJ, editors. Anesthesia for otolaryngologic surgery. London: Cambridge University Press; 2012. p. 58–82.

7. Mason RA, Fielder CP. The obstructed airway in head and neck surgery. Anaesthesia 1999;54(7):625–8.

8. Artime C, Hagberg C. Airway management. In: Miller RD, editor. Miller's anesthesia. 8th edition. Philadelphia: Churchill Livingstone/Elsevier; 2014. p. 1647–83.

9. Rosenblatt W, Ianus AI, Sukhupragarn W, et al. Preoperative endoscopic airway examination (PEAE) provides superior airway information and may reduce the use of unnecessary awake intubation. Anesth Analg 2011;112(3):602–7.

10. Woodall N, Frerk C, Cook TM. Can we make airway management (even) safer?– lessons from national audit. Anaesthesia 2011;66(Suppl 2):27–33.

11. Hohn A, Kaulins T, Hinkelbein J, et al. Awake tracheotomy in a patient with stridor and dyspnoea caused by a sizeable malignant thyroid tumor: a case report and short review of the literature. Clin Case Rep 2017;5(11):1891–5.

12. Rosenblatt WH. The airway approach algorithm: a decision tree for organizing preoperative airway information. J Clin Anesth 2004;16(4):312–6.

13. Benumof JL. Management of the difficult adult airway. With special emphasis on awake tracheal intubation. Anesthesiology 1991;75(6):1087–110.

14. Rosenstock CV, Thogersen B, Afshari A, et al. Awake fiberoptic or awake video laryngoscopic tracheal intubation in patients with anticipated difficult airway management: a randomized clinical trial. Anesthesiology 2012;116(6):1210–6.

15. Reed AP. Preparation of the patient for awake flexible fiberoptic bronchoscopy. Chest 1992;101(1):244–53.

16. Walsh ME, Shorten GD. Preparing to perform an awake fiberoptic intubation. Yale J Biol Med 1998;71(6):537–49.

17. Rosenblatt W, Artime C. Management of the difficult airway for general anesthesia in adults. 2019. Available at: UpToDate.com. Accessed March 21, 2019.

18. Iseli TA, Iseli CE, Golden JB, et al. Outcomes of intubation in difficult airways due to head and neck pathology. Ear Nose Throat J 2012;91(3):E1–5.

19. Kaplan MB, Hagberg CA, Ward DS, et al. Comparison of direct and video-assisted views of the larynx during routine intubation. J Clin Anesth 2006;18(5): 357–62.

20. Aziz MF, Dillman D, Fu R, et al. Comparative effectiveness of the C-MAC video laryngoscope versus direct laryngoscopy in the setting of the predicted difficult airway. Anesthesiology 2012;116(3):629–36.

21. Jungbauer A, Schumann M, Brunkhorst V, et al. Expected difficult tracheal intubation: a prospective comparison of direct laryngoscopy and video laryngoscopy in 200 patients. Br J Anaesth 2009;102(4):546–50.

22. Roy S, Basañez I, Alexander R. Rigid bronchoscopy. In: Hagberg CA, Artime CA, Aziz MF, editors. Hagberg and Benumof's airway management. 4th edition. Philadelphia: Elsevier; 2018. p. 517–24.

23. Artime C. Flexible fiberoptic intubation. In: Hagberg CA, Artime CA, Daily WH, editors. The difficult airway: a practical guide. Oxford (England): Oxford University Press; 2013. p. 97–108.

24. Sofferman RA, Johnson DL, Spencer RF. Lost airway during anesthesia induction: alternatives for management. Laryngoscope 1997;107(11 Pt 1):1476–82.

25. Boyce JR, Peters GE, Carroll WR, et al. Preemptive vessel dilator cricothyrotomy aids in the management of upper airway obstruction. Can J Anaesth 2005;52(7): 765–9.

26. Kaufman MR, Alfonso KP, Burke K, et al. Awake vs sedated tracheostomies: a review and comparison at a single institution. Otolaryngol Head Neck Surg 2018; 159(5):830–4.

27. Sagiv D, Nachalon Y, Mansour J, et al. Awake tracheostomy: indications, complications and outcome. World J Surg 2018;42(9):2792–9.

28. Fang CH, Friedman R, White PE, et al. Emergent Awake tracheostomy–The five-year experience at an urban tertiary care center. Laryngoscope 2015;125(11):2476–9.

29. Rashid A, Raj B, Stoddart A. Repeat percutaneous dilatational tracheostomy in an awake and unintubated patient. Acta Anaesthesiol Scand 2007;51(3):378–9.

30. Asai T, Koga K, Vaughan RS. Respiratory complications associated with tracheal intubation and extubation. Br J Anaesth 1998;80(6):767–75.

31. Peterson GN, Domino KB, Caplan RA, et al. Management of the difficult airway: a closed claims analysis. Anesthesiology 2005;103(1):33–9.

32. Cavallone LF, Vannucci A. Review article: extubation of the difficult airway and extubation failure. Anesth Analg 2013;116(2):368–83.

33. Mathew JP, Rosenbaum SH, O'Connor T, et al. Emergency tracheal intubation in the postanesthesia care unit: physician error or patient disease? Anesth Analg 1990;71(6):691–7.

34. Rothaar RC, Epstein SK. Extubation failure: magnitude of the problem, impact on outcomes, and prevention. Curr Opin Crit Care 2003;9(1):59–66.

35. Difficult Airway Society Extubation Guidelines Group, Popat M, Mitchell V, Dravid R, et al. Difficult Airway Society Guidelines for the management of tracheal extubation. Anaesthesia 2012;67(3):318–40.

36. Artime CA, Hagberg CA. Tracheal extubation. Respir Care 2014;59(6):991–1002 [discussion: 1002–5].

37. Russo SG, Goetze B, Troche S, et al. LMA ProSeal for elective postoperative care on the intensive care unit: a prospective, randomized trial. Anesthesiology 2009; 111(1):116–21.

38. Fujii Y, Toyooka H, Tanaka H. Cardiovascular responses to tracheal extubation or LMA removal in normotensive and hypertensive patients. Can J Anaesth 1997; 44(10):1082–6.

39. Nair I, Bailey PM. Use of the laryngeal mask for airway maintenance following tracheal extubation. Anaesthesia 1995;50(2):174–5.

40. Ellard L, Brown DH, Wong DT. Extubation of a difficult airway after thyroidectomy: use of a flexible bronchoscope via the LMA-classic. Can J Anaesth 2012; 59(1):53–7.

Anesthetic Management of the Narrowed Airway

Daniel John Doyle, MD, PhD, DPhil[a,b,*], Anastasios G. Hantzakos, MD, PhD, MHA, FEBORL[b,c]

KEYWORDS

- Airway fire • Airway stents • Balloon dilatation • Laser airway surgery
- Microdebridement • Narrowed airway • Tracheal stenosis

KEY POINTS

- Some causes of airway narrowing include postintubation tracheal stenosis, airway tumors, hematomas, infections, foreign bodies, and airway edema.
- Endoscopic treatment of airway narrowing includes balloon dilatation, stent placement, laser ablation, microdebridement, and other techniques. Both rigid bronchoscopy and flexible bronchoscopic techniques may be used.
- Jet ventilation is frequently used in the management of many airway procedures, especially when the presence of an endotracheal tube would interfere with the surgery.
- Anesthesia in airway surgery is commonly achieved using a total intravenous technique such as a propofol infusion in conjunction with a remifentanil infusion.
- An airway fire is potentially lethal complication that may occur during airway surgery, especially with airway laser procedures or during tracheotomy surgery.

INTRODUCTION

Narrowed or stenotic airways are frequently encountered in otolaryngologic practice (**Fig. 1**).[1] This article is intended as an overview of the numerous anesthetic and safety considerations in dealing with such cases. By necessity this presentation is only a broad overview, and the reader interested in more details will need to consult other papers in this issue as well as some of the references provided herein. In addition, this article focuses on upper airway problems. For example, bronchial asthma can be viewed as a cause of lower airway narrowing, but its treatment is not discussed here. Nor is the management of Obstructive Sleep Apnea,

Disclosure Statement: The authors have nothing to disclose.
[a] Department of General Anesthesiology, Cleveland Clinic Abu Dhabi, Abu Dhabi, UAE;
[b] Cleveland Clinic Lerner College of Medicine, Cleveland, OH, USA; [c] Department of Otolaryngology and Head and Neck Surgery, Cleveland Clinic Abu Dhabi, Box 112412, Abu Dhabi, UAE
* Corresponding author. Department of Anesthesia, Cleveland Clinic Abu Dhabi, Box 112412, Abu Dhabi, UAE.
E-mail address: djdoyle@hotmail.com

Otolaryngol Clin N Am 52 (2019) 1127–1139
https://doi.org/10.1016/j.otc.2019.08.010
0030-6665/19/© 2019 Elsevier Inc. All rights reserved.

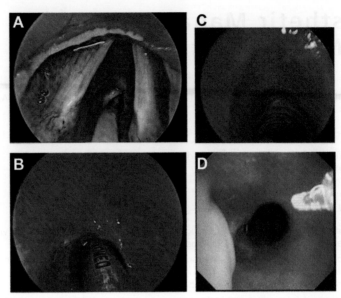

Fig. 1. (*A*) [*Upper left*] Patient with Grade 3 idiopathic subglottic stenosis, as seen with a 0° Hopkins laryngeal telescope. Suspension laryngoscopy and jet ventilation were used. (*B*) [*Lower left*] Microdebridement of the same subglottic stenosis shown on Figure 1a. (*C*) [*Upper right*] Endoscopic image of the same patient in Figure 1a and b after completion of the microdebridement. (*D*) [*Lower right*] Treatment of subglottic stenosis with a flexible CO_2 laser system (Lumenis Duo Flexilase). The laser fiber is passed through the working channel of a flexible endoscope.

which is arguably a form of narrowed airway (the narrowing commonly occurring at the velopharynx).[2]

CAUSES OF AIRWAY NARROWING AND AIRWAY STENOSIS

Some of the more common causes of airway narrowing and stenosis are listed in **Boxes 1–3**. Some of these are genuine airway emergencies (eg, pediatric epiglottitis, obstructing foreign bodies, hematomas compressing the airway), whereas some can be handled more electively (as with most cases of tracheal stenosis). Note that patients presenting with stridor always require immediate clinical attention.

Although in some of these cases tracheal intubation will be necessary to establish a definitive airway, in some other cases less invasive interventions may suffice. For instance, patients with an edematous airway following prolonged airway instrumentation (eg, with a rigid bronchoscope) may have been treated with steroids (eg, dexamethasone 8 mg intravenously [IV]) and topical dilute epinephrine (eg, epinephrine 1:100,000 in 1–2 mL increments) but may need additional time for a full therapeutic effect. In such cases heliox may be administered as an effective temporizing measure. This is discussed further in Case Study 1. In some of these patients noninvasive biphasic positive airway pressure ventilation would be another temporizing measure.

It is worth emphasizing that excessive airway cuff pressures during tracheal intubation is a frequently unrecognized source of airway stenosis. Tracheal tube cuff

---

Box 1
A list of some of the more common causes of airway narrowing and stenosis

- Tracheal stenosis (postintubation, GERD-related, post–lung transplantation, idiopathic)
- Tumors (intraluminal, extraluminal/extrinsic compression)
- Hematomas (eg, hematomas following thyroid surgery, carotid artery surgery, or trauma to the neck)
- Infections (eg, epiglottitis, Ludwig angina, retropharyngeal abscess)
- Foreign body aspiration (such items are frequently retrieved via rigid bronchoscopy)
- Airway edema (post–airway instrumentation, pregnancy, hereditary angioedema, smoke and hot gas inhalation)

Abbreviation: GERD, gastroesophageal reflux disease.

---

pressures are easily measured with a cuff pressure manometer and should ordinarily be between 20 and 30 cm H_2O. Excessive cuff pressures can result in tracheal stenosis, tracheal necrosis, and even tracheal rupture as a result of diminished blood flow to tracheal mucosa. This hypothesized ischemic injury then produces healing fibrosis months or even years later.[3]

ENDOSCOPIC MANAGEMENT

Airway endoscopy plays an important role in the diagnosis and treatment of airway tumors and especially to manage benign and malignant airway stenoses.[4,5] More recently, endoscopic techniques have also been developed to treat end-stage emphysema, manage air leaks from bronchopleural fistulae, and treat intractable asthma via thermoablation.[5–7]

The frequency of central airway obstruction is increasing, paralleled with the increasing incidence of lung cancer. The development of endoscopic methods has allowed for less invasive management of these patients, with balloon dilation, laser therapy, microdebridement, and airway stenting as some of the options available to patients with central airway obstruction.

Box 2
Some common and uncommon airway management techniques in managing the narrow or stenotic airway

- Spontaneous ventilation in conjunction with an inhalation anesthetic induction
- Spontaneous ventilation in conjunction with an airway adjunct such as an OPA or NPA (following induction of anesthesia)
- Conventional positive pressure ventilation with an SGA (eg, i-gel) or ETT (wide bore preferred) or rigid bronchoscope
- Jet ventilation (see text)
- Positive/negative pressure ventilation via Ventrain system (see text)
- Extracorporeal membrane oxygenation (see text)

Abbreviations: ETT, endotracheal tube; NPA, nasopharyngeal airway; OPA, oropharyngeal airway; SGA, supraglottic airway.

Box 3
Helpful hints to bear in mind in dealing with patients with a narrow airway

- Patients presenting with stridor always command immediate attention. Although tracheal intubation is often required in such settings, less invasive interventions (eg, heliox administration) are sometimes appropriate as a temporizing measure.

- A joint review of available computed tomographic scans and airway videos by the anesthesiologist and surgeon together immediately before the procedure will help confirm the joint management plan.

- Although an inhalation induction is commonly recommended in pediatric patients with epiglottitis, this technique is usually unsatisfactory in adult patients with severe tracheal stenosis. (When an inhalational induction is attempted in such patients the induction is often slow and complicated by apneic episodes, hypoxemia, and a need to use bag-mask positive pressure ventilation to rescue the patient.)

- When using rigid bronchoscopy, avoid inhalational agents such as sevoflurane because they are not delivered reliably (scope going in and out) and they pollute the room terribly. Use a propofol infusion in conjunction with a remifentanil infusion instead. Muscle relaxation is usually needed.

- In addition, when using rigid bronchoscopy, it is frequently helpful to pack the oropharynx with saline soaked gauze to reduce the leak to manageable levels. (Leave a portion of each gauze outside the mouth as a reminder.)

- In cases where deep neuromuscular blockade is needed until the very end of the procedure, reversal with sugammadex is often preferable to using neostigmine and glycopyrrolate.

BALLOON DILATATION

Flexible bronchoscopic balloon dilatation is often used alone or in conjunction with other therapies to dilate narrowed airways.[8–10] As an example, the CRE Pulmonary Balloon Dilatation Catheter series from Boston Scientific is designed to endoscopically dilate narrowed airways via a 2.8 mm bronchoscope working channel. An excellent endoscopic video illustrating the technique is available at https://s3.amazonaws.com/prod.csurgeries.com/modify/csurgeries_20130923035501.mp4.

LASER AIRWAY SURGERY

Laser airway surgery can be done in 1 of 2 major ways: with a laser-safe endotracheal tube in place or using total intravenous anesthesia (TIVA) with jet ventilation. In the former situation volatile anesthetics may be used but conventional endotracheal tubes must be avoided, as they are flammable. (For a dramatic video showing an endotracheal tube [ETT] set on fire by a carbon dioxide [CO_2] laser see https://www.youtube.com/watch?v=zl8OAxpf9es). The lasers used in such settings are often CO_2 lasers and Nd-YAG lasers, depending on the clinical situation. The CO_2 laser offers precise cutting with a fine zone of coagulation that helps reduce surgical bleeding, whereas light emitted from an Nd-YAG laser can be transmitted through flexible quartz fibers that can be used in conjunction with a fiberoptic bronchoscope.

Surgical lasers release great energy and can cause unintended tissue damage as well as operating room fires. This concern is discussed later in this article. An additional concern with laser airway surgery is the smoke plume, which may be a vector for viral spread in some cases. As a result, continuous smoke evacuation is mandatory.[11,12]

MICRODEBRIDEMENT

Microdebrider bronchoscopy is a new airway surgical technique that allows for precise removal of obstructing airway tissue. The technique is done under general anesthesia with either a rigid bronchoscope or (less commonly) a suspension laryngoscope, with the microdebrider typically operating at 1000 to 3000 rpm.[13,14] One important advantage of the technique is the avoidance of the complications of thermal techniques (eg, lasers or argon plasma coagulation) such as airway fires.

STENTS

Silicone and self-expandable metallic airway stents (SEMS) are the main stent types used in airway management.[15,16] Although silicone stents are often the preferred modality because they are easily repositioned, SEMS are frequently used in cases of airway wall malacia or stenosis, especially in the context of malignancy. SEMS have the advantage over silicone stents of a lower migration rate, thinner wall construction (allowing for greater cross-sectional airway diameter), and conformation to irregular airways. Although SEMS placement is ordinarily achieved endoscopically with relative ease, removal can be very difficult. Indications for SEMS removal include excessive or recurrent granulation, stent failure or fracture, infection, mucous plug formation, stent migration, or completion of successful treatment. Complications during stent removal may include pneumothorax; tracheal, bronchial, laryngeal, or pulmonary artery injury; and airway obstruction during or following stent removal.

JET VENTILATION

Jet ventilation is frequently used in the management of many otolaryngologic procedures, especially when the presence of an endotracheal tube would interfere with the surgery, such as with the treatment of some tracheal stenosis. Two techniques are available: (1) use of a simple hand-held device and (2) use of an automatic jet ventilator system. In both cases 100% oxygen delivery is possible but many automated jet ventilators have blenders to mix oxygen and air to reduce the Fio_2. Although the Venturi effect causes entrainment of room air with the resulting gas mixture of less than 100%, it is prudent to use a gas mixture less than 100% and to ensure the Fio_2 is less than 30% during laser surgery. In the case of hand-held devices, the operator starts operation with a driving pressure set to about around 20 psi (in adults) and provides manually delivered jets of a little less than 1 second duration delivered approximately 10 to 20 times a minute. In most cases the jet ventilation apparatus is attached to an anterior commissure laryngoscope or other type of otolaryngologic laryngoscope via a screw attachment to provide supraglottic ventilation. The main means of determining that ventilation is adequate is to watch the chest rise with each delivered jet pulse. For safety reasons the driving pressure should be adjusted down to the minimum needed to achieve adequate chest excursions. Note that obese individuals require higher driving pressures to achieve adequate chest excursions as compared with lean patients.

In the case of an automatic jet ventilator system, a commercial product such as that provided by the Acutronic Company may be used to provide infraglottic ventilation. This is usually achieved in conjunction with an infraglottic ventilation catheter. Note that the ventilation rates for infraglottic automatic jet ventilation systems are usually much higher (in the range of 100 per minute and upwards) than for the supraglottic manual jet ventilation systems mentioned earlier (which typically operate in the range of 10–20 per minute).

Most complications associated with the use of jet ventilation are due to use of a high pressure of the delivered gas, and barotrauma leading to pneumothorax, pneumomediastinum, or other problems can result from the high pressures used, which can run as high as 50 psi (which is equal to 3500 cm H_2O pressure). This is particularly true if gas trapping due to an inadequate expiratory pathway takes place.

ANESTHETIC TECHNIQUE

The following anesthetic technique will serve as a rough guide to most cases involving conventional or bronchoscopic surgery used to manage a narrowed airway and is based on the clinical judgment of the surgeon and anesthesiologist who believe the narrowed airway is sufficient to permit anesthetic induction. If there is any doubt, an awake fiberoptic intubation with a small endotracheal tube or awake tracheostomy should be performed.

After the induction of general anesthesia with propofol and muscle relaxation achieved with a paralytic such as rocuronium, anesthesia is commonly maintained using a TIVA technique such as a propofol infusion delivered at an initial rate of 100 mcg/kg/min in conjunction with a remifentanil infusion delivered at an initial rate of 0.1 mcg/kg/min. These infusions are then adjusted based on the factors such as the hemodynamics and the depth of anesthesia as guided by clinical findings and (commonly, but not always) by electroencephalographic analysis.

In some centers it is common to add 1 mg of remifentanil to 500 mg (50 mL) of propofol and treat the combination as "superpropofol," delivering it in a single syringe at an initial rate of 100 mcg/kg/min of propofol. When 100 mcg/kg/min of propofol is delivered in this scheme, the resulting rate of remifentanil infusion is then 0.2 mcg/kg/min. This arrangement has the advantage that only a single syringe pump is needed but has the disadvantage that the 2 infusions cannot be independently adjusted. Also if this scheme is used the pump should be correctly labeled to indicate the medications being infused. This should also be mentioned with any transfer of care that may occur during a procedure.

PREVENTION AND MANAGEMENT OF AIRWAY FIRES

An airway fire is potentially lethal complication that may occur during airway surgery, especially with airway laser procedures or during tracheotomy surgery. Case study 2 provides an example. For any fire to occur the triad of fuel (eg, ETT, drapes, sponges), oxidizer (O_2 or N_2O), and an ignition source (eg, laser or electrocautery) is needed. Consequently, in at-risk situations oxygen concentrations should be kept to a minimum, and nitrous oxide (which also supports combustion) should also be avoided. Further details are provided in the American Society of Anesthesiologists Operating Room Fire Algorithm (**Fig. 2**).

In general, airway fires call for the immediate removal of the ETT, turning the oxygen/nitrous oxide sources off and flooding the field with saline from a prefilled 50 mL syringe. Although conventional wisdom holds that airway fires require the immediate removal of the ETT, it should be recognized that there are some situations (eg, patients who were very difficult to intubate in the first place) where removal of the ETT would in all likelihood result in irreversible loss of the airway. Clinicians in such a setting face a particularly challenging choice: leave the tube in place and risk fire-related injury to the patient or remove the tube and risk loss of the airway.[17]

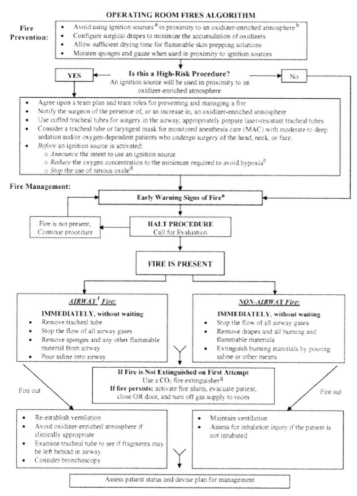

OPERATING ROOM FIRES ALGORITHM

Fig. 2. American Society of Anesthesiologists Operating Room Fire Algorithm. [a] Ignition sources include but are not limited to electrosurgery or electrocautery units and lasers. [b] An oxidizer-enriched atmosphere occurs when there is any increase in oxygen concentration above room air level and/or the presence of any concentration of nitrous oxide. [c] After minimizing delivered oxygen, wait a period of time (eg, 1–3 min) before using an ignition source. For oxygenation patients, *reduce* supplemental oxygen delivery to the minimum required to avoid hypoxia. Monitor oxygenation with pulse oximetry, and if feasible, inspired, exhaled, and/or delivered oxygen concentration. [d] After stopping the delivery of nitrous oxide, wait a period of the (eg, 1–3 min) before using an ignition source. [e] Unexpected flash, flame, smoke, or heat; unusual sounds (eg, a "pop," "snap", or "foomp") or odors; unexpected movement of drapes, discoloration of drapes or breathing circuit; unexpected patient movement or complaint. [f] In this algorithm, airway fire refers to a fire in the airway or breathing circuit. [g] A CO_2 fire extinguisher may be used on the patient if necessary. (*From* Apfelbaum JL, Caplan RA, Barker SJ, Connis RT, Cowles C, Ehrenwerth J, Nickinovich DG, Pritchard D, Roberson DW, Caplan RA, Barker SJ, Connis RT, Cowles C, de Richemond AL, Ehrenwerth J, Nickinovich DG, Pritchard D, Roberson DW, Wolf GL. Practice advisory for the prevention and management of operating room fires: an updated report by the American Society of Anesthesiologists Task Force on Operating Room Fires. Anesthesiology. 2013 Feb;118(2):271-90; with permission.)

Lasers and Unique Considerations

When lasers are in use it is prudent to remember that lasers used in surgery produce high amounts of optical energy. To warn everyone of this danger, one should place warning signs outside the operating room and opaque coverings should be placed on any operating room windows to prevent stray laser beams from exiting. Safety goggles should also be used; these are specific to each laser type.

An even greater danger during laser airway surgery with an ETT in place is an airway fire, so laser-safe ETTs are necessary. For instance, the Mallinckrodt Laser-Flex ETT is a stainless-steel spiral wound tube with 2 PVC cuffs that are often filled with diluted methylene blue to allow early detection of a cuff leak. With 2 cuffs the distal cuff maintains a seal if the proximal one is ruptured. Other popular tubes are the Sheridan LASER-TRACH and the Rusch Lasertubus, both which use an embossed copper foil covering a rubber tube. When used, the minimum acceptable Fio$_2$ should be used and a 50-cc saline-filled syringe should be immediately available to use as an improvised fire extinguisher.

Finally, note that the presence of high oxygen concentrations near the patient's face can promote fires in this region, so delivering supplementary oxygen by face mask or nasal cannula requires special care. ANSI standard Z136.3 (Safe Use of Lasers in Health Care Facilities) provides additional relevant information.

THE VENTRAIN SYSTEM

Mechanical ventilation of patients is usually carried out using a conventional diameter (eg, 6–8 mm internal diameter [ID]) low-resistance cuffed tracheal tube inserted into the patient's trachea. There are circumstances, however, where this arrangement is inappropriate. For instance, as noted earlier, with some forms of laryngeal surgery a narrow-diameter high-resistance catheter (eg, Hunsaker catheter) driven by a high-pressure gas source is used instead in order to offer the surgeon an unimpeded view of the glottis. Another situation is the "cannot intubate, cannot oxygenate/ventilate" (CICO/V) emergency, where percutaneous transtracheal jet ventilation via a very narrow bore high-resistance catheter is sometimes recommended as a life-saving procedure. In all these cases expiration during ventilation occurs passively, but a recently introduced new technology now exists that supports active expiration via a narrow-bore catheter. Known as the Ventrain system, the device allows for full ventilation via a mere 2 to 3 mm catheter, even in fully obstructed airways, using active expiration based on the Bernoulli Principle. The result is a system of ventilation that avoids extreme intrapulmonary pressures and the associated pulmonary (baro)trauma that sometimes plagues jet ventilation. As such the device is shown to be a lifesaver of babies and adults, providing full ventilation in CICO/V situations.[18–21]

As shown in **Figs. 3** and **4**, Ventrain is a compact, manually operated hand-held ventilator specifically designed for ventilation through narrow-bore (eg, 2–3 mm ID) catheters such as the Tritube narrow-bore cuffed endotracheal tube (**Fig. 5**). As noted earlier, what makes the Ventrain unique in comparison to other ventilation systems is its application of the Bernoulli principle to apply suction (as opposed to mere passive gas flow) during the expiratory phase of ventilation. This breakthrough in ventilator design allows for minute ventilation rates in excess of 7 L/min with relatively modest oxygen flows of 15 L/min and using catheters with internal diameters as narrow as 2 mm via any route of airway access.[22]

In CICO/V situations the Ventrain system has shown value during upper airway surgery by improving surgical exposure and avoiding the potential need for

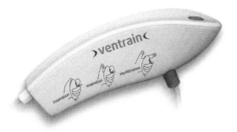

Fig. 3. The Ventrain device. This simple-to-operate manual ventilator is operated using one's thumb and index finger. It features active expiration based on the Bernoulli principle, allowing ventilation through small-bore tubes. In addition to inspiratory (positive pressure) and expiratory (negative pressure) modes of operation, an equilibration (safety) mode is available where no significant positive or negative pressure is present at the tip of the attached ventilation catheter. (*Courtesy of* Ventinova Medical, Eindhoven, The Netherlands; with permission.)

tracheostomy. Borg and colleagues[23] were the first to describe the use of Ventrain during upper airway surgery, chronicling the use of the Ventrain during a laryngoscopy procedure in a stridorous patient suffering from an exophytic glottic tumor. A 2-mm ID transtracheal catheter was inserted into the cricothyroid membrane under local anesthesia and connected to the Ventrain using an oxygen flow of 15 L per minute. General anesthesia was then induced and the patient ventilated via the Ventrain at 15 breaths per minute (inspiration for 2 seconds, then expiration for 2 seconds). The procedure, which lasted 15 minutes, was uneventful and resulted in biopsy samples that allowed for the patient's condition to be more reliably evaluated.

Onwochei and colleagues[24] described a 2-stage technique to manage airway obstruction and avoid a surgical tracheostomy in a 49-year-old woman who suffered from "postradiotherapy laryngeal fixation and transglottic stenosis" and had a pharyngeal stricture in need of dilation. Their technique involved awake fiberoptic intubation,

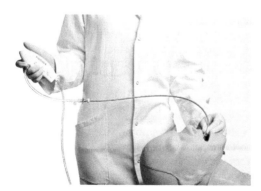

Fig. 4. Ventrain used in conjunction with a small-bore airway catheter such as those used to exchange endotracheal tubes or those used to assist with tracheal extubation. In addition to providing a means to facilitate reintubation, such airway catheters can also be used with the Ventrain to maintain ventilation and oxygenation until a definitive airway is established. (*Courtesy of* Ventinova Medical, Eindhoven, The Netherlands; with permission.)

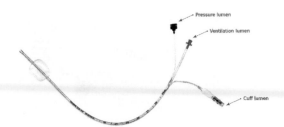

Fig. 5. The Tritube is a narrow-bore cuffed ETT with inner and outer diameters 2.4 mm and 4.4 mm, respectively. A Murphy eye is featured at the distal end. The ventilation lumen is attached to the Ventrain, whereas an inflatable cuff seals the airway. A pressure measurement lumen permits continuous intratracheal pressure measurements. This device may be useful in both elective and emergency airway settings. (*Courtesy of* Ventinova Medical, Eindhoven, The Netherlands; with permission.)

followed by the transtracheal insertion of a Cricath flexible 2-mm needle cricothyrotomy catheter, with ventilation using the Ventrain system. Similarly, Fearnley and colleagues[25] described the elective use of the Ventrain for upper airway obstruction in a patient with post-radiation fibrosis that had previously prevented passive expiration during attempted high-frequency jet ventilation.

Kristensen and colleagues[26] used the Ventrain in conjunction with a special 2.4-mm ID cuffed tracheal tube (Tritube) allowing intratracheal pressure monitoring in 7 ENT surgical patients. In all patients, adequate ventilation with intratracheal pressures between 5 and 20 cm H_2O was performed. The investigators noted that the combination of Ventrain with Tritube provided an "unprecedented view of the intubated airway during oral, pharyngeal, laryngeal or tracheal procedures" and even noted that the techniques has the "potential to replace temporary tracheostomy, jet-ventilation or extra-corporal membrane oxygenation in selected patients." In their series, Kristensen and colleagues also mention that one patient was transported to the postanesthetic care unit (PACU) with a Tritube in place (with the cuff deflated) and was subsequently uneventfully extubated.

Where a hand-operated technique is burdensome, clinicians may wish to use the new and Conformité Européenne-approved automatic ventilator Evone instead, allowing ventilation through the thin and cuffed Tritube. Product details are available at https://www.ventinovamedical.com/evone/. Barnes and Enk[27] and Schmidt and colleagues[28] have recently executed useful studies awaiting publication dealing with the Evone that will interest those seeking further information.

EXTRACORPOREAL MEMBRANE OXYGENATION IN THE MANAGEMENT OF THE CRITICAL AIRWAY

In desperate cases, extracorporeal membrane oxygenation (ECMO) may occasionally be used in managing the critical airway. As an example, Holliday and Jackson[29] reported on the use of ECMO to support a severely intoxicated patient with a life-threatening airway obstruction preventing adequate oxygenation and ventilation despite the presence of an ETT used to secure the airway. Fiberoptic bronchoscopy revealed a large tracheal food bolus situated beyond the ETT. With ECMO instituted, the obstructing food bolus was removed via rigid bronchoscopy under controlled conditions. A recent review by Hoetzenecker and colleagues[30] provides a review of the published ECMO experience in relation to airway surgery in both in adult and pediatric patients.

CASE STUDY 1: USE OF HELIOX

A 58-year-old female patient needed surgery for recurrent head and neck cancer. Because of her pathology, she was particularly difficult to intubate via a flexible bronchoscope. On extubation the patient became severely stridorous despite being wide awake and undergoing full reversal of neuromuscular blockade. Treatment included 2 IV doses of 8 mg dexamethasone (1 administered preextubation), 2 doses of nebulized racemic epinephrine (0.5 mL of 2.25% epinephrine added to 2.5 mL saline), and assisted mask ventilation with the patient sitting up at 60°, but despite this, the patient did not improve and was becoming exhausted. As reintubation would have been even more difficult than it had been earlier, a surgical airway was considered the only option.

The use of heliox, mixture of helium (70%) and oxygen (30%), delivered using a nonrebreathing face mask at 10 L/min saved the patient from needing a surgical airway. Approximately 5 to 10 breaths of heliox and the stridor vanished, and the patient's work of breathing became much more manageable. The patient was then brought to the PACU with full monitoring and with a heliox tank in tow. She was then weaned off the heliox over several hours.

Case Study 1 Discussion

Airway obstructing conditions producing stridor may be modeled as breathing through an orifice (a situation where a tube length is smaller than its radius). Under such conditions, the approximate flow across the orifice varies inversely with the square root of the gas density. This is in contrast to the usual laminar flow situation during breathing, where gas flow varies inversely with gas viscosity. Note that although the viscosity values for helium and oxygen are similar, their densities are very different (density @ 20°C: air 1.293 g/L; nitrogen 1.250 g/L; oxygen 1.429 g/L; helium 0.178 g/L). In summary, the low density of helium allows it to play an important role in the management of some forms of airway obstruction associated with gas turbulence, and heliox for delivery with a nonrebreathing face mask should be readily available in every operating room suite.

CASE STUDY 2: AIRWAY FIRE

The following case reported by Salaria and colleagues[31] illustrates the complexity that may be involved in managing an airway fire. A 79-year-old man with severe aortic stenosis and multiple other comorbidities underwent an endoluminal minimally invasive mitral valve repair, aortic valve replacement, and MAZE procedure with a stormy postoperative course complicated by respiratory failure and necessitating an elective tracheostomy. One hundred percent oxygen was provided for preoxygenation before the tracheal incision. When the surgeon began to use monopolar electrocautery, "a 3-cm flame arose from the tracheal incision site." In response, the field was flooded with saline, the ETT removed, the Fio_2 decreased to room air, and the patent reintubated via the tracheal incision. Once the situation was stable, video laryngoscopy and fiberoptic visualization "revealed edematous, red, and inflamed mucosa in the right upper lobe and middle lobe bronchus" as well as "mild edema and red, inflamed mucosa" of the supraglottic structures. In the intensive care unit (ICU), a postoperative chest computed tomography "revealed bilateral patchy, nodular air space opacities and ground glass opacities with right perihilar bronchial thickening," whereas "repeat fiberoptic bronchoscopy demonstrated blackened tracheal mucosa distal to the tracheal tube" with all 3 segments of the right upper lobe heavily charred. Despite fastidious care in the ICU that included "inhaled heparin every 8 hours,

N-acetylcysteine, and albuterol" as well as daily bronchoscopy to clear mucous impaction, the patient ultimately died after developing multiorgan dysfunction.

Case Study 2 Discussion

Here the authors agree to what the investigators said about their case.

"The cutting action of bipolar cautery generates lower temperatures, less tissue damage, and avoidance of sparks. In our case, the precipitating event was the use of monopolar diathermy to control bleeding in the presence of ventilation with 100% FiO_2."

REFERENCES

1. Cooper JD. Tracheal injuries complicating prolonged intubation and tracheostomy. Thorac Surg Clin 2018;28(2):139–44.
2. Finkelstein Y, Wolf L, Nachmani A, et al. Velopharyngeal anatomy in patients with obstructive sleep apnea versus normal subjects. J Oral Maxillofac Surg 2014; 72(7):1350–72.
3. Feng TR, Ye Y, Doyle DJ. Critical importance of tracheal tube cuff pressure management. World J Anesthesiol 2015;4(2):10–2.
4. Murgu SD, Egressy K, Laxmanan B, et al. Central airway obstruction: benign strictures, tracheobronchomalacia, and malignancy-related obstruction. Chest 2016;150(2):426–41.
5. Walters DM, Wood DE. Operative endoscopy of the airway. J Thorac Dis 2016; 8(Suppl 2):S130–9.
6. Paradis TJ, Dixon J, Tieu BH. The role of bronchoscopy in the diagnosis of airway disease. J Thorac Dis 2016;8(12):3826–37.
7. Ong PG, Debiane LG, Casal RF. Recent advances in diagnostic bronchoscopy. J Thorac Dis 2016;8(12):3808–17.
8. Wright CD. Nonoperative endoscopic management of benign tracheobronchial disorders. Thorac Surg Clin 2018;28(2):243–7.
9. Sharma SD, Gupta SL, Wyatt M, et al. Safe balloon sizing for endoscopic dilatation of subglottic stenosis in children. J Laryngol Otol 2017;131(3):268–72.
10. Ozturk K, Erdur O, Sofiyev F, et al. Noninvasive treatment of acquired subglottic stenosis. J Craniofac Surg 2016;27(5):e492–3.
11. Mowbray N, Ansell J, Warren N, et al. Is surgical smoke harmful to theater staff? a systematic review. Surg Endosc 2013;27(9):3100–7.
12. Ulmer BC. The hazards of surgical smoke. AORN J 2008;87(4):721–34 [quiz: 735].
13. Lunn W, Garland R, Ashiku S, et al. Microdebrider bronchoscopy: a new tool for the interventional bronchoscopist. Ann Thorac Surg 2005;80(4):1485–8.
14. Casal RF, Iribarren J, Eapen G, et al. Safety and effectiveness of microdebrider bronchoscopy for the management of central airway obstruction. Respirology 2013;18(6):1011–5.
15. Cooper JD. Use of silicone tubes in the management of complex airway problems. Thorac Surg Clin 2018;28(3):441–7.
16. Tjahjono R, Chin RY-K, Flynn P. Tracheobronchial stents in palliative care: a case series and literature review. BMJ Support Palliat Care 2018;8(3):335–9.
17. Chee WK, Benumof JL. Airway fire during tracheostomy: extubation may be contraindicated. Anesthesiology 1998;89(6):1576–8.

18. Willemsen MGA, Noppens R, Mulder ALM, et al. Ventilation with the Ventrain through a small lumen catheter in the failed paediatric airway: two case reports. Br J Anaesth 2014;112(5):946–7.
19. Escribá Alepuz FJ, Alonso García J, Cuchillo Sastriques JV, et al. Emergency ventilation of infant subglottic stenosis through small-gauge lumen using the ventrain: a case report. A A Pract 2018;10(6):136–8.
20. Wahlen BM, Al-Thani H, El-Menyar A. Ventrain: from theory to practice. Bridging until re-tracheostomy. BMJ Case Rep 2017;2017. https://doi.org/10.1136/bcr-2017-220403.
21. Heuveling DA, Mahieu HF, Jongsma-van Netten HG, et al. Transtracheal use of the cricath cannula in combination with the ventrain device for prevention of hypoxic arrest due to severe upper airway obstruction: a case report. A A Pract 2018;11(12):344–7.
22. Hamaekers AEW, Borg PAJ, Enk D. Ventrain: an ejector ventilator for emergency use. Br J Anaesth 2012;108(6):1017–21.
23. Borg PAJ, Hamaekers AEW, Lacko M, et al. Ventrain® for ventilation of the lungs. Br J Anaesth 2012;109(5):833–4.
24. Onwochei DN, El-Boghdadly K, Ahmad I. Two-stage technique used to manage severe upper airway obstruction and avoid surgical tracheostomy: a case report. A A Pract 2018;10(5):118–20.
25. Fearnley RA, Badiger S, Oakley RJ, et al. Elective use of the Ventrain for upper airway obstruction during high-frequency jet ventilation. J Clin Anesth 2016;33:233–5.
26. Kristensen MS, de Wolf MWP, Rasmussen LS. Ventilation via the 2.4 mm internal diameter Tritube® with cuff - new possibilities in airway management. Acta Anaesthesiol Scand 2017;61(6):580–9.
27. Barnes T, Enk D. Ventilation for low dissipated energy achieved using flow control during both inspiration and expiration. Trends in Anaesthesia and Critical Care 2019;24:5–12.
28. Schmidt J, Günther F, Weber J, et al. Flow-controlled ventilation (FCV) in the perioperative setting – an observational two-centre first-in-human study. Eur J Anaesth 2019;36(5):327–34.
29. Holliday T, Jackson A. Emergency use of extracorporeal membrane oxygenation for a foreign body obstructing the airway. Crit Care Resusc 2010;12(4):273–5.
30. Hoetzenecker K, Klepetko W, Keshavjee S, et al. Extracorporeal support in airway surgery. J Thorac Dis 2017;9(7):2108–17.
31. Salaria ON, Suthar R, Abdelfattah S, et al. Perioperative management of an airway fire: a case report. A A Pract 2018;10(1):5–9.

19. Villcormeer MGA, Koppens R, Hazee AHJ, et al. Ventilation via the Ventrain through a small lumen catheter in the failed paediatric airway: two case report. Br J Anaesth 2014;113(6):935-7.

20. Escriva Alepuz FJ, Alberti Garcia J, Gutierrez Serrano JV, et al. Emergency ventilation of infant subglottic stenosis through small catheter using the Ventrain. A case report. A A Pract 2018;10(4):136-8.

21. Yamin BM, Al-Thani H, El-Menyar A. Ventrain: from theory to practice. Bridging until re-tracheostomy. BMJ Case Rep 2017;2017. https://doi.org/10.1136/bcr-2017-220403.

22. Hamaekers AE, Borg PAJ, Enk D. Ventrain: an ejector ventilator for emergency use. Br J Anaesth 2012;108(6):1017-21.

23. Berg PAJ, Hamaekers AEW, Fakle M, et al. Ventrain for ventilation of the lungs. Br J Anaesth 2012;108(6):1024-5.

26. Kristensen MS, de Wolf MWP, Rasmussen LS. Ventilation via the 2.4 mm internal diameter Tritube with continued severe subglottic stenosis: a airway management. Acta Anaesthesiol Scand 2017;61(6):626-9.

27. [illegible]

28. [illegible]

29. [illegible]
Anaesthesia 2015;70(10):1207-51.

30. Halliday T, Jackson A. Emergency use of cricothyroid membrane oxygenation before or during difficult airway. Dublin.

31. Bourdeau [illegible], Naguib M, Kamath A, et al. Expiration close suction in airway surgery. J [illegible] Dis 2017;9(12):1694-7.

32. Sabina GH, Sahar A, Abdelrahim S, et al. Retrograde management of an airway [illegible] airway [illegible] A A Pract 2018;10(10):1-3.

Critical Care and Postoperative Management of the Head and Neck Patient

Bharat Akhanda Panuganti, MD[a], Philip A. Weissbrod, MD[a],
Jaspreet Somal, MBBS[b],*

KEYWORDS

- Postoperative management • Head and neck • Critical care • Trauma

KEY POINTS

- Head and neck surgical patients, at times, can represent a challenging population to manage in the intensive care unit postoperatively.
- Close interaction between the critical care and surgical teams, awareness of potential surgery-specific complications, and utilization of protocol-driven care can reduce risk of morbidity significantly in this population and enhance outcomes.
- Given the relative complexity of otolaryngologic surgery and the unique risk that head and neck pathologies can pose to patient airway, breathing, and circulation, these collective circumstances warrant detailed discussion in the interest of minimizing patient morbidity and mortality.

INTRODUCTION

Quality improvement has become a ubiquitous mandate in health care, owing to the significant cost of medical errors. The Institute of Medicine landmark report, "To Err Is Human," estimated that approximately 98,000 deaths occurred in the United States due to preventable medical errors. In 2008, it was estimated that medical errors cost the United States $19.5 billion.[1] Although mechanisms to improve patient care continue to be innovated, a common underlying theme in the broader effort to deliver quality care is the importance of interdisciplinary collaboration. Anesthesiologists and otolaryngologists share a unique clinical relationship characterized by a synergistic expertise in airway management. This opportunity for collaboration continues in the postoperative period, where cooperation between otolaryngology and critical care services is necessary for safe and effective patient care. Given the relative complexity of otolaryngologic surgery, and the unique risk

Disclosure: None.
[a] Department of Surgery, Division of Otolaryngology–Head and Neck Surgery, University of California San Diego, 200 West Arbor Drive, MC# 8895, San Diego, CA 92103, USA;
[b] Department of Anesthesiology and Critical Care, University of California San Diego, San Diego, CA, USA
* Corresponding author.
E-mail address: jsomal@ucsd.edu

that head and neck pathologies can pose to patient airway, breathing, and circulation, these collective circumstances warrant detailed discussion in the interest of minimizing patient morbidity and mortality.

GENERAL POSTOPERATIVE CONSIDERATIONS IN HEAD AND NECK SURGERY PATIENTS

Venous Thromboembolism Prophylaxis

Deep vein thrombosis (DVT) and pulmonary emboli (PE) are common complications in surgical patients. For general surgical procedures, the rates of DVT and PE formation without chemical prophylaxis have been reported to be between 15% and 30% and 0.2% and 0.9%, respectively.[2] On average, postoperative venous thromboembolisms (VTEs) increase hospital length of stay by more than 5 days and are associated with a 6.56% excess mortality rate in patients undergoing oncologic procedures.[3] Although the risk of VTE among general surgery, trauma, and orthopedic patients is well established, protocols dictating the use of VTE prophylaxis in otolaryngology are less definitive. Studies estimating the incidence of VTE after otolaryngology procedures have reported much lower rates for DVT (approximately 0.3%); the risk is higher among patients undergoing oncologic head and neck procedures (approximately 0.6%).[4] The lower overall incidence of VTEs after otolaryngology procedures is attributable to the sizable proportion of patients undergoing low-morbidity surgeries that do not impede early mobility or require lengthy inpatient recovery. Although longer duration of hospitalization is associated with increased VTE risk, no studies have established a projected length-of-stay cutoff to consider prophylaxis. Risk stratification to identify subpopulations with a relative predisposition for thromboembolic events can permit clinicians to prioritize thromboprophylaxis for patients in whom risk of bleeding is outweighed by reduction in VTE risk. Bahl and colleagues[5] report on their use of the Caprini risk assessment model, which considers 40 weighted risk factors (eg, family history of VTE, obesity, and history of malignancy) in order to stratify head and neck surgery patients by VTE risk (**Fig. 1**). Their analysis of 3498 hospitalized, postoperative otolaryngology patients failed to reveal a difference in overall incidence of VTE with (1.2%) and without (1.3%) chemoprophylaxis. A subanalysis of high-risk patients (Caprini score >8), however, revealed that the incidence of VTE was 10.7% with chemoprophylaxis and 18.3% for patients without it. Of clinical import, they noted a statistically significant difference in bleeding complications (3.5% vs 1.2%) incidence of postoperative bleeding complication with and without chemoprophylaxis associated with chemoprophylaxis; lastly, prophylaxis was found to be of significant benefit in patients who underwent microvascular reconstruction (7.7% vs 2.1% incidence of VTE without chemoprophylaxis).[4] A recent practice guideline pertaining VTE prophylaxis after otolaryngologic surgery delineated chemoprophylaxis guidelines based explicitly on patient Caprini scores, suggesting that patients with a score of 5 to 6 should be considered for chemoprophylaxis; patients with a score of 7 or higher were recommended to receive dual prophylaxis, including both chemoprophylaxis and mechanical prophylaxis.[6]

In summary, thromboprophylaxis should be strongly considered in head and neck surgery patients with high-risk comorbid conditions (eg, limited mobility, malignancy, obesity, free flap reconstruction, and long duration of hospitalization). Appropriate risk stratification may help prevent bleeding events in cases of low relative probability of VTE.

Prophylactic Antibiotics

Preoperative antibiotic prophylaxis is often administered in otolaryngology given the common instrumentation of the upper aerodigestive tract. The precise indications

Each Risk Factor Represents 1 Point
☐ Age 41–60 y
☐ Minor surgery planned
☐ History of prior major surgery (<1 mo)
☐ Varicose veins
☐ History of inflammatory bowel disease
☐ Swollen legs (current)
☐ Obesity (BMI >25)
☐ Acute myocardial infarction
☐ Congestive heart failure (<1 mo)
☐ Sepsis (<1 mo)
☐ Serious lung disease incl. pneumonia (<1 mo)
☐ Abnormal pulmonary function (COPD)
☐ Medical patient currently at bed rest
☐ Other risk factors_____

Each Risk Factor Represents 2 Points
☐ Age 60–74 y
☐ Arthroscopic surgery
☐ Malignancy (present or previous)
☐ Major surgery (>45 min)
☐ Laparoscopic surgery (>45 min)
☐ Patient confined to bed (>72 h)
☐ Immobilizing plaster cast (<1 mo)
☐ Central venous access

Each Risk Factor Represents 5 Points
☐ Elective major lower extremity arthroplasty
☐ Hip, pelvis, or leg fracture (<1 mo)
☐ Stroke (<1 mo)
☐ Multiple trauma (<1 mo)
☐ Acute spinal cord injury (paralysis)(<1 mo)

Each Risk Factor Represents 3 Points
☐ Age over 75 yr
☐ History of DVT/PE
☐ **Family history of thrombosis**[a]
☐ Positive factor V Leiden
☐ Positive prothrombin 20210A
☐ Elevated serum homocysteine
☐ Positive lupus anticoagulant
☐ Elevated anticardiolipin antibodies
☐ Heparin-induced thrombocytopenia
☐ Other congenital or acquired thrombophilia
If yes:
Type_____
[a]most frequently missed risk factor

For Women Only (Each Represents 1 Point)
☐ Oral contraceptives or hormone replacement therapy
☐ Pregnancy or postpartum (<1 mo)
☐ History of unexplained stillborn infant, recurrent spontaneous abortion (≥3), premature birth with toxemia or growth-restricted infant

Total Risk Factor Score ☐

Fig. 1. Thrombosis risk factor assessment used by clinicians to determine a patient's Caprini score. BMI, body mass index; COPD, chronic obstructive pulmonary disease; incl., including. (*From* Caprini JA. Thrombosis Risk Assessment as a Guide to Quality Patient Care. *Dis Mon.* 2005;51(2-3):70-78; with permission.)

for and duration of postoperative prophylaxis, however, are subjects of debate. Postoperative prophylactic antibiosis is not indicated in clean cases (eg, thyroidectomies) due to the low overall risk of surgical site infection (SSI). Prophylactic antibiotics offered after clean-contaminated procedures, however, have been shown to affect SSI risk (reduction from 24%–78% to 5.8%–38% of procedures with extended prophylaxis).[7] Given the polymicrobial colonization of the upper aerodigestive tract, including by gram-negative and anaerobic species, the consensus is that prophylaxis should be more extensive than a single-agent cephalosporin (eg, cefazolin). Langerman and colleagues[8] completed a retrospective multi-institution analysis comparing ampicillin-sulbactam, clindamycin, cefazolin and metronidazole, and cefazolin alone and noted an approximate two-thirds risk reduction in odds of SSI (odds ratio [OR] 0.28; 95% CI, 0.13–0.61) when ampicillin-sulbactam was administered for 24 hours postoperatively. Antibiotics, however, should not be offered for more than 24 hours postoperatively. Vila and colleagues[9] completed a meta-analysis of antibiotic prophylaxis in clean-contaminated head and neck surgeries and found that the pooled relative risk (RR) of wound infections in patients receiving 1 day versus 5 days of prophylaxis was 0.98 (95% CI, 0.58–1.61).

Free flap reconstructive cases are commonly complicated by SSIs (13.3%), with microvascular reconstruction reported as an independent risk factor for SSIs (Yarlagadda and colleagues 2016[10]). A systematic review assessing prophylaxis in clean-contaminated head and neck procedures with free flap reconstruction initially found that longer duration of postoperative prophylactic antibiosis was associated with a reduced SSI risk (RR 1.56%; 95% CI, 1.13–2.14). A post hoc multivariate analysis meant to evaluate the effect of antibiotic type on SSI risk, however, found that although duration of prophylactic antibiosis was not an independent risk factor for SSIs, the use of clindamycin was associated with a significant increase in likelihood of SSI risk (RR 2.85; 95% CI, 1.95–4.17). Another study revealed that clindamycin was associated with an approximate 4-fold increase in risk for SSI (OR 3.784; 95% CI, 1.367–10.47) after free tissue transfer cases (Pool and colleagues 2016[11]). As the untoward effects of clindamycin as an alternative to β-lactam antibiotics have become more apparent, otolaryngologists have started to avoid its use in the periop-erative setting. A second-generation or third-generation cephalosporin with extended aerobic gram-negative coverage can be considered in cases of a true penicillin allergy (Jethwa and Khariwala 2017[12]). In summary, prophylactic antibiosis should be offered for only 24 hours after clean-contaminated otolaryngologic cases and should be prioritized in patients who underwent free flap reconstruction.

Nutrition and Swallowing

The perioperative management of head and neck surgery patients often requires a multidisciplinary approach (eg, nutrition, speech language pathology [SLP], physical therapy, and respiratory therapy), given the significant potential functional morbidity associated with otolaryngologic pathologies and the procedures meant to treat them. Feeding, in particular, is an important consideration in the postoperative setting and can be restricted due to neuromuscular dysfunction, anatomic alteration, or pres-ence of mucosal incision. As much as 52% of the head and neck cancer population is malnourished at the time of diagnosis, owing to obstruction, trismus, odynophagia, and/or sensory impairment.[13] Nutritional status has even been cited as an indepen-dent prognosticator of survival among head and neck cancer patients.[14] In general, larger surgical defects are associated with greater deficits in both speech and swal-lowing; patients with extirpative defects requiring bulky, afunctional microvascular free flaps can be associated with even poorer swallowing outcomes. Aspiration is a possible complication after an ablative procedure at virtually any level within the upper aerodigestive tract, affecting anything from bolus formation and propulsion to airway protection. As such, early consultation with SLP for bedside swallow evaluation can improve early swallow outcomes and minimize the risk of pneumonia. The modified barium swallow study is often recommended by SLPs as part of their evaluation, which is performed by administering radioactive contrast by mouth under fluoroscopy. The purposes of the modified barium swallow study are to identify the location and extent of dysfunction, to determine the relative safety of swallowing, and to guide subsequent rehabilitative strategies in terms of textural and positional recommendations. In some institutions, flexible endoscopic evaluation of swallowing can provide similar informa-tion. Gastrostomy tube placement can be considered when a feeding conduit is required for more than 2 weeks; a nasogastric tube can be considered as an alterna-tive feeding mechanism for shorter durations.

General Concepts in Extubation After Head and Neck Surgery

According to the American Society of Anesthesiologists (ASA) Closed Claims Project study, claims related to difficult airway management outside the operating theater are more likely to lead to fatal outcomes than those occurring within the operating room.[15] The head and neck surgical population, in particular, presents a level of airway complexity due to altered postoperative anatomy and tissue changes related to chemoradiation (eg, edema and fibrosis), making reintubation after failed extubation tenuous.

Rates of reintubation have been reported to be between 0.7% and 11.1% after maxillofacial and major neck surgeries.[16,17] Protocols meant to aid clinicians facilitate successfully timed extubation in high-risk patients have been published. The 2003 ASA guidelines broadly suggest that a preformulated extubation strategy include (1) consideration of the relative merits of awake extubation versus extubation before the return of consciousness, (2) evaluation of clinical factors that may produce an adverse impact on ventilation after the patient has been extubated, (3) the formulation of an airway management plan to be implemented if the patient is unable to maintain adequate ventilation after extubation, and (4) consideration of the short-term use of a device that can serve as a guide for expedited reintubation.[18] The Difficult Airway Society guidelines offer a comprehensive checklist defining the high-risk extubation population and sequential steps to prevent and to manage complicated or premature extubation.[19]

The plan for extubation should be jointly decided between the otolaryngologist and the anesthesiologist, with consideration for the difficulty of the initial intubation (eg, potentially complicated by poor neck extension, an anteriorly oriented larynx, edema associated with preexisting infection, or history of radiation), the duration of the surgery, and the probability of postoperative swelling or bleeding. Surgical instrumentation of the upper aerodigestive tract often results in bleeding retained in the pharynx; thorough suction with an orogastric tube prior to extubation can help deter aspiration events and help reduce the probability of laryngospasm. Other procedure-specific considerations, including the possibility of vocal cord paralysis after thyroidectomy, and fundamental changes to the airway anatomy (eg, total laryngectomy) that may affect conditions for reintubation are separately discussed later.

PROCEDURE-SPECIFIC CONSIDERATIONS IN HIGH-RISK HEAD AND NECK SURGERY PATIENTS IN THE POSTOPERATIVE SETTING
Free Tissue Transfer

Large oncologic resections in the head and neck can have significant consequences for a patient speech, swallowing, and appearance, for which the versatility of microvascular free tissue reconstruction is uniquely effective in minimizing. Although a variety of local rotation and pedicled flaps (eg, pectoralis major myofascial flap) are available for use, they are inherently limited by a plane of rotation, restricted bulk, and/or the inability to include bone in the reconstruction. More than 40 donor sites for free tissue transfer to the head and neck have been described, although the radial forearm, fibula, rectus, and jejunal free flaps account for 92% of all free flaps used for head and neck reconstruction.[20] Microvascular reconstruction is commonly considered for composite defects of the oral cavity (eg, after tongue, cheek, or floor of mouth is extirpated with a segment of mandible), extensive pharyngoesophageal defects, or large scalp or cervicofacial defects (**Fig. 2**). The osteocutaneous fibula free flap has become the mainstay for oromandibular reconstruction at many institutions, due to the 25 cm of bone available for harvest; the excess length is particularly important when bony reconstruction is required in multiple dimensions.

Carefully guided postoperative management of free flap patients is integral to avoid the morbidity associated with free flap failure. More than 95% of free flap compromise occurs within the first 72 postoperative hours.[21] Compared with arterial insufficiency, venous thrombosis is the more common anastomotic complication.[22] Mechanical stress exerted by a hematoma and vascular kinking due to flap geometry also are potential causes of failure. Given the inherently tenuous nature of fresh vascular

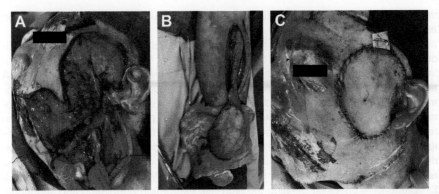

Fig. 2. (*A*) Radical parotidectomy, including wide local excision of overlying skin resulting in a significant left facial soft tissue defect. (*B*) Harvest of a radial forearm fasciocutaneous free flap demonstrating both the soft tissue and vascular pedicle meant for reconstruction. (*C*) Radial forearm free flap after inset and closure of former left facial soft tissue defect.

anastomoses, free flap patients often are admitted to the intensive care unit (ICU) for close nursing and physician care for at least the first 24 hours postoperatively. At the authors' institution, the flap is monitored every hour for the first 24 hours, every 2 hours for the following 24 hours, and every 4 hours for the remaining duration of the admission. Monitoring protocols vary by institution and surgeon. Physical examination remains 1 cornerstone of free flap monitoring. This includes visual inspection of the free flap, making note of progressive swelling and/or color changes (duskiness, mottling, and ecchymosis), evaluation of temperature (a well-perfused flap is generally warm), turgor (a firm, stiffened flap may suggest underlying congestion or hematoma), and assessment of capillary refill. Scratching or pricking the flap with a small hypodermic needle to evaluate the timing and color of bleeding is a useful maneuver when flap vitality is uncertain. Slightly delayed, bright red bleeding is seen in well-perfused flaps. The absence of bleeding and brisk egress of dark, deoxygenated blood (venous congestion) are signs concerning for a threatened flap. In cases of the free flap vascular pedicle that is accessible, Doppler monitoring is a valuable adjunctive technique. Emittance of a robust, triphasic Doppler signal, corresponding to rapid antegrade flow during systole, transient reversal of flow during early diastole, and slow antegrade flow during late diastole, is a reassuring sign of viability. Early recognition of a threatened flap is essential to permit successful surgical salvage, because prolonged ischemia can cause indelible damage. Hyodo and colleagues[23] reported that the mean postoperative, re-exploration time for successful salvage was 1.3 days in their case series compared with 3.9 days for failed salvages.

Transoral Oropharyngeal Surgery

Transoral laser microsurgery and transoral robotic surgery represent 2 approaches to treat diseases of the oropharynx, larynx, and hypopharynx without the morbidity of an open approach, while maintaining favorable oncologic outcomes. Transoral surgery for the oropharynx has become increasingly commonplace, owing to the increasing numbers of palatine tonsil and base of tongue squamous cell carcinomas related to human papillomavirus infections. Robotic surgery, in particular, has gained increasing popularity due its additional benefits of binocular, high-definition, 3-D microscopy aided by tremor-free hand controls and 6° of freedom provided by the transoral robotic arms. Given wide laryngopharyngeal accessibility and significantly improved range of motion, head and neck surgeons have been able to perform diagnostic and therapeutic oropharyngectomies, including wide sampling of both the lingual and palatine tonsils in the cases of head and neck squamous cell carcinomas with unknown primary tumors.

The oropharynx is well vascularized, receiving its arterial blood supply from multiple branches of the external carotid artery. Bleeding rates after transoral oropharyngectomy procedures are reported to be between 3% and 10%, which are approximately commensurate with reported bleeding incidences after nononcologic, routine palatine tonsillectomies (2%–8%).[24] When an oropharyngectomy is completed with a concomitant neck dissection, branches of the external carotid (eg, lingual, facial, and/or superior thyroid arteries) often are ligated prophylactically, although a recent study failed to reveal a statistically significant difference in hemorrhage with intraoperative ligation.[24] Despite no difference in overall rates of hemorrhage, ligation has been reported to reduce the incidence of catastrophic events.[25] Oropharyngeal hemorrhage is a potentially catastrophic complication, given the inability to effectively pack the oropharynx in an awake patient and the threat of airway compromise/asphyxiation. Major bleeding events warrant prompt airway securement, which, in cases of significant oropharyngeal hemorrhage, may necessitate an awake, emergent tracheostomy or cricothyrotomy. Patients with an existing tracheostomy should either immediately have their cuff inflated or have their tracheostoma intubated with a cuffed endotracheal tube. Once the airway is secure, the oropharynx can be immediately packed off and the bleeding controlled intraoperatively. In some circumstances, the culprit vessel has spasmed shut after airway securement. Consultation with interventional radiology to consider endovascular embolization should be made when intraoperative localization of the bleeding vessel is difficult.

Epistaxis and Cerebrospinal Fluid Leak After Endoscopic Sinus Surgery

Endoscopic sinus surgery (ESS) is one of the most commonly performed procedures in otolaryngology. Major complications, including cerebrospinal fluid (CSF) leak (0.17%–0.5%), orbital injury (0.07%), and epistaxis requiring a transfusion (0.76%), are rare but potentially devastating sequelae of sinus surgery.[26,27] Endoscopic instrumentation of the sinonasal vault usually is performed for the treatment of chronic or recurrent acute rhinosinusitis or for the extirpation of skull base or sinonasal tumors. Intraoperative computed tomography (CT) image guidance, which allows precise instrument localization relative to a preoperative CT scan, frequently is used, given the proximity of the paranasal sinuses to important vasculature (internal carotid artery in the sphenoid sinus and branches of the ophthalmic artery lining the skull base) and other vital anatomy (skull base, orbit, and the optic nerve accessible via the sphenoid sinus).

CSF leak occurs after inadvertent penetration of bone and dura lining the anterior skull base, including the cribriform plate (most common site for iatrogenic CSF leak), leading to a direct communication between the intracranial and sinonasal cavities. Leaks identified intraoperatively are fully exposed and repaired, usually with a combination of bioadhesives, biologic autografts or homografts, and free or pedicled tissue flaps. A vast majority of leaks (91%–97%) are repaired successfully endoscopically without further sequelae.[28] Effective, primary leak repair is essential, because the incidence of meningitis with persistent CSF rhinorrhea has been reported to be as high as 22%.[29] Although postoperative admission is not strictly necessary, a short observation stay may be considered to confirm successful leak repair and to monitor for neurologic changes that may be associated with massive pneumocephalus or delayed intracranial hemorrhage. Postoperative lumbar drain placement to reduce intracranial pressures and prophylactic antibiotic use after iatrogenic CSF leak repair are not routinely indicated, although antistaphylococcal antibiotics usually are administered to ESS patients with endonasal packing in place. A recent meta-analysis reviewing 508 cases found that the use of perioperative lumbar drains did not have a significant effect on CSF leak recurrence rates after endoscopic repair, although some clinicians consider its use in cases of a high-flow leak characterized by direct transmission from a cistern or ventricle.[30]

Regarding antibiotic use, a Cochrane review investigating the value of prophylactic antibiotics in patients with basilar skull fractures (with or without rhinorrhea) found that prophylactic antibiosis failed to affect the incidence of meningitis, all-cause mortality, or meningitis-related mortality.[31] The patient population in this study, however, was distinct from patients with acute/chronic sinusitis where a CSF leak has occurred in an infected field. The use of perioperative antibiotics should be a decision based on clinical judgment. In the postoperative setting, patients must abide closely to CSF leak precautions, including avoidance of straining (stool softeners should be liberally administered) or strenuous physical activity; use of open-mouthed coughing or sneezing; sleeping with head-of-bed elevation to 15° to 30° (angle of inclination reduces CSF pressure at the basal cisterns); and minimizing caffeine intake. Clinicians should be suspicious of a recurrent CSF leak if a patient reports frank, clear rhinorrhea (usually unilateral) and/or postnasal drip with a salty or metallic character.

The nose and the paranasal sinuses have a robust vascular supply, derived mostly from branches of the sphenopalatine artery. A branch of the sphenopalatine artery, the posterior septal branch, is the most common site for postoperative bleeding after ESS. Although a certain amount of bloody nasal drainage postoperatively is expected, any patient presenting with brisk epistaxis after ESS should be evaluated endoscopically. Conservative measures, including liberal oxymetazoline application through the bleeding naris and use of inflatable, nonabsorbable packing with concomitant resorbable hemostatic preparations (eg, thrombin-gelatin hemostatic matrix), frequently are unsuccessful in the postoperative setting. As indicated previously, post-ESS epistaxis is commonly the result of damage to a posterior vessel, which may necessitate the use of a posterior nasal pack, including a Foley catheter to occlude the nasal choana and a nonabsorbable nasal pack anterior to the Foley balloon for widespread compression. Surgical intervention as the primary treatment of posterior epistaxis is associated, however, with shorter hospital stay, higher success rate, and an overall cost savings of $1846.[32] Surgical intervention should be strongly considered when a posterior nasal pack is required for the acute management of epistaxis and/or if the epistaxis is iatrogenic. Patients admitted to the hospital with recently treated epistaxis should practice precautions similar to those for patients admitted with a history of a CSF leak.

Tracheostomy

Tracheostomy is another commonly performed procedure by head and neck surgeons; more than 100,000 tracheostomies are performed annually in the United States, and approximately one-third of patients requiring prolonged ventilation receive a tracheostomy.[33,34] There is significant ongoing debate, however, regarding the optimal time to consider a tracheostomy in an intubated patient. The oft-referenced 1989 *Chest* consensus guidelines recommended translaryngeal ventilation when respiratory support was anticipated for less than 10 days and a tracheostomy when it was expected for more than 21 days.[35] A recent meta-analysis found that early tracheostomy (performed within 7 days of endotracheal intubation) was associated with a significant reduction in mean ICU length of stay (9.13 days), although no differences were found in hospital mortality or incidence of ventilator-associated pneumonia.[36] A large multicenter, prospective randomized trial involving ventilated patients in the United Kingdom, the Tracheostomy Management in Critical Care trial, failed to realize differences in length of ICU or total hospital stay, incidence of pneumonia and 30-day all-cause mortality between 455 patients who underwent an early tracheostomy (before 4 days) and 454 patients who underwent a late tracheostomy (7 days or later).[34]

Although there is continued uncertainty regarding some of the immediate benefits of early tracheostomy procedures, of particular concern to otolaryngologists is the laryngotracheal morbidity of endotracheal intubation. Unfortunately, there is considerable reported variability in the absolute duration and risk factors affiliated with endotracheal tube–related laryngotracheal injury. A study by Santos and colleagues[37] reported on risk factors associated with laryngeal injury after endotracheal intubation for longer than 3 days, finding that 97% of subjects had some degree of laryngeal injury (ranging from mild edema or erythema to vocal fold immobility) and that duration of intubation and the concomitant presence of a nasogastric tube were associated risk factors. Another study found that limiting endotracheal intubation to 9.1 days with an endotracheal tube up to a size 8 (10.9-mm outer diameter) was safe without increasing the risk of immediate laryngeal injury (Colton House and colleagues 2011[38]). Contrarily, a commonly cited study by Halum and colleagues[39] established that endotracheal intubation for more than 1 week was associated with 2.42 times the odds (95% CI, 0.81–7.89) of airway stenosis, also indicating that obesity (9.9% incidence of airway stenosis in this population) and use of bigger endotracheal tubes (>7.5) were robust predictors.

Posterior glottic stenosis (PGS), in particular, represents a dreaded and difficult-to-treat complication of endotracheal intubation, caused by damage to the interarytenoid mucosa and arytenoid cartilages, ultimately resulting in interarytenoid fibrosis, contracture, and even cricoarytenoid joint fixation. Although the extent of PGS can be variable, a classification system described by Bogdasarian and Olson stratified the severity of PGS to 4 types (type 1 representing simple synechiae and type 4 representing posterior commissure stenosis with bilateral ankylosis).[40] A 1984 prospective study of 200 intubated patients found that the incidence of PGS was 5% in patients intubated between 5 days and 10 days and 12% in those intubated between 11 days to 24 days.[41] A more recent appraisal of 36 PGS patients found that each additional day of intubation was associated with a 21% increase in odds of PGS and that comorbid diabetes mellitus was associated with 888% increased odds (OR 8.88; 95% CI, 2.27–34.72) of PGS.[42] Although not typically found to be an acute ICU-related risk given the time stenosis takes to develop, it is an important consideration when making decisions about long-term ventilatory options.

Prolonged endotracheal intubation is also a risk factor for subglottic stenosis (SGS)—a study by Manica and colleagues[43] revealed that for every 5 additional days of intubation, there was a 50.3% increase in the odds of developing SGS. Although there is semantic disagreement regarding the optimal timing of a tracheostomy, the broad consensus is that early tracheostomy when prolonged endotracheal intubation needs are anticipated is useful to avoid laryngotracheal morbidity and improve patient comfort.

There are several important complications of tracheostomies to consider in the postoperative setting. The overall rate of complications for patients undergoing tracheotomies is 3.2%.[44] Tracheoinnominate fistula (TIF) represents a highly uncommon (0.1%–1.0% of all tracheostomies) but life-threatening complication that occurs with peak incidence between the first and second postoperative weeks and is the result of tracheal ulceration from sustained tracheostomy tube irritation.[45] Although the majority of fistulae formation occurs at the level of the tracheostomy tube cuff, ulceration can also initiate due to pressure from the elbow or tip of the cannula. Patients initially may present with a lower-volume, self-limited sentinel bleed, which has been reported to occur approximately 50% of the time.[46] Immediate management of TIF includes immediate over-inflation of the tracheostomy balloon to compress the bleeding innominate vessel, which is successful in approximately 85% of cases. If hemorrhage continues despite balloon over-inflation, a cuffed orotracheal tube should be advanced past the level of tracheostoma, and finger pressure should be applied to the innominate artery through the stomal opening. After airway stabilization, the patient should be immediately mobilized to the operating room; TIF mortality without surgical exposure and innominate arterial ligation is 100%.[45]

Unplanned decannulation represents another potentially devastating post-tracheostomy adverse event and is reported to occur in 4.2 of 1000 tracheostomy days.[47] Accidental decannulations in patients with a mature tracheostoma (>7 days old) and normal cervical anatomy usually are benign occurrences, assuming the tracheostomy is replaced in a timely fashion prior to closure of the stoma. Decannulations in the more immediate postoperative setting, particularly in patients with poor underlying respiratory reserve, a proximal airway obstruction, or abnormal neck anatomy, can be sources of significant morbidity and/or mortality. At the authors' institution, the phalanges of the tracheostomy tubes are sutured to the peristomal skin and maintained until the fifth to seventh postoperative days, in order to preserve more durable tube fixation until stomal maturation. Moreover, in some cases, an inferiorly based Bjork flap (trap-door flap created in the anterior tracheal wall inferior to the tracheotomy) is reflected anteriorly and sewn to the inferior aspect of the stoma, in order to enhance access to the tracheotomy in cases of decannulation.

Thyroidectomy

Thyroidectomies are generally a well-tolerated procedure, with a low overall incidence of postoperative morbidity (5%–7%).[48] Recurrent laryngeal nerve injury (temporary or permanent) complicates between 0.4% and 7.2% of thyroidectomy procedures. The recurrent laryngeal nerve innervates most of the intrinsic laryngeal musculature; damage to it can impair or paralyze ipsilateral vocal cord movement. Intraoperative recurrent laryngeal nerve monitoring has been introduced as an adjunct meant to aid in successful identification and preservation of the recurrent nerves, although its value in mitigating the risk of permanent nerve dysfunction is dubious.[49] Even unilateral recurrent laryngeal nerve injury, and associated unilateral vocal cord paresis or paralysis, can have important functional sequelae. For example, laryngeal penetration or aspiration has been reported in approximately one-third of patients with unilateral vocal cord immobility.[50] Bilateral recurrent laryngeal nerve injury is an exceedingly rare phenomenon (0.1% incidence reported at a high-volume endocrine surgical unit). In cases of bilateral midline cord fixation, patients present with severe respiratory distress that might require emergent tracheostomy. Early recognition of this complication, particularly after completion thyroidectomies wherein the contralateral nerve is known preoperatively to be paralyzed, should prompt expeditious airway management.

Studies have demonstrated that up to 37% of patients after a total or completion thyroidectomy with parathyroid gland preservation suffer from at least temporary hypoparathyroidism, usually due to ischemic insult from manipulation of the parathyroid glands or their vascular pedicle. Although 70% of patients who undergo total thyroidectomy with parathyroid gland conservation revert to a euparathyroid state within 2 months of surgery, supplementation in the immediate postoperative setting may still be necessary.[51] Both routine and selective calcium and vitamin D supplementation after total or completion thyroidectomies have been advocated, and both parathyroid hormone (PTH) and calcium (either ionized or total serum) levels have been proposed to guide the extent of supplementation. A study by Sywak and colleagues reported that a postoperative PTH of 20 ng/L had a 96% sensitivity in predicting hypocalcemia but reported maximal specificity with a threshold of 3 ng/L; the investigators recommended an intermediate PTH threshold of 10 ng/L to determine whether patients would be supplemented with calcium alone or in conjunction with vitamin D.[52] Other investigators have advocated inclusion of vitamin D in any situation postoperatively wherein calcium supplementation is initiated, because production of 1,25-dihydroyvitmain D (which stimulates intestinal absorption and promotes bone remodeling) is impaired in hypoparathyroidism. Calcitriol is the biologically active form of vitamin D, of which standard postoperative dosing is 0.25 μg administered twice daily. Standard calcium supplementation typically requires 1 g to 2 g of elemental calcium 3 times daily. Supplementation is often inadequate, in which case additional calcium and/or vitamin D may be necessary.[53] For patients with milder symptoms of neuromuscular irritability (eg, perioral paresthesia and extremity numbness/tingling) and calcium concentrations greater than 7.5 mg/dL (after adjustment for serum albumin), the frequency of oral calcium supplementation can be increased to 4 times daily and the total calcitriol dose can be increased. Intravenous calcium supplementation, in the form of calcium gluconate or calcium chloride (preferred less due to the potential for local tissue necrosis with extravasation) should be considered in cases of severe hypocalcemia (less than 7.5 mg/dL) with significant symptoms (seizures and electrocardiogram changes).[54] Intravenous calcium supplementation should be considered until stable serum calcium concentrations are sustained with oral supplementation alone.

Thyroid hormone supplementation also should be initiated after total or completion thyroidectomy procedures. Synthetic T4 (levothyroxine) is the most common form of long-term supplementation (1.7 mg/kg oral dosing), although synthetic T3 (liothyronine) supplementation is started when radioactive iodine is anticipated as an adjuvant therapy.

Total Laryngectomy

The total laryngectomy procedure refers to the surgical removal of the larynx, interrupting the traditional orotracheal respiratory pathway and instead diverting airflow through a cervical tracheastoma. Common indications include locally advanced laryngeal or hypopharyngeal tumors, chronic aspiration, and laryngeal chondroradionecrosis. Advanced hypopharyngeal tumors may require a laryngopharyngectomy procedure, wherein both the pharynx and cervical esophagus are mobilized with the larynx during the extirpation.

After a total laryngectomy, orotracheal intubation and supplemental oxygen delivered either by nose or mouth are no longer viable options. Rapid airway securement, if necessary, can be accomplished via the patient's tracheastoma. Total laryngectomy patients usually are admitted to the ICU postoperatively, given their aphonia and elevated risk of airway loss (eg, pneumonia and stomal edema or dehiscence) in the immediate postoperative period. Patients often leave the operating room with a laryngectomy tube to maintain stomal patency and reduce crusting associated with the tracheocutaneous anastomosis; these devices are not meant to be used for mechanical ventilation.

There is some variation in clinical practice regarding the initiation of oral feeding after a total laryngectomy. A 1989 survey of US surgeons revealed that 84% of practitioners waited until after the seventh postoperative day to begin feeds by mouth, in the interest of allowing sufficient time for the pharyngeal suture line to heal.[55] Indeed, pharyngocutaneous fistulae (PCF) have been reported to complicate as many as 70% of salvage total laryngectomies, prolonging hospital stay and interfering with wound healing. More importantly, chronic exposure of the neck contents to saliva and refluxate can be corrosive; the presence of a PCF is a risk factor for carotid blowouts.[56] A 2008 study published by Aswani and colleagues, however,[57] found no difference in the incidence of PCF formation between patients who were fed early and in delayed fashion. Moreover, use of a pectoralis major myofascial overlay flap, at least in the high-risk, salvage setting, has been shown to reduce the risk of PCF formation by 22%.[58] PCF have been reduced by adherence to a postoperative protocol, recently published by Li and colleagues.[59] The protocol mandates (1) thyrotropin testing in all patients with a history of head and neck radiation and initiation of 100 μg daily of levothyroxine in any patient with a history of chemoradiation, (2) a standardized 2-layer pharyngeal closure, (3) pedicled pectoralis muscular onlay flap over the pharyngeal closure in any patient with a history of chemoradiation, and (4) 2 doses of postoperative antibiotics.[59]

Other Common Otolaryngologic Postoperative Complications

Chyle leak
Chyle leakage from iatrogenic thoracic duct injury is a known complication after 2% to 8% of cervical lymphadenectomies, in particular those in the inferior left neck.[60,61] The thoracic duct is situated in the left neck, draining lymph from the left body and infradiaphragmatic right body, and usually drains into the internal jugular vein near its confluence with the subclavian vein. Chyle is composed of both lymphatic fluid and lipid-containing chylomicrons absorbed from the gastrointestinal system. Whereas chylomicrons are formed from the metabolism of long-chain fatty acids by bile salts, more water-soluble medium-chain fatty acids are absorbed directly into the hepatic portal system, bypassing the lymphatic system.

When a chyle leak is identified intraoperatively, the ends of the traumatized thoracic duct are identified and ligated; the addition of fibrin-based preparations to the wound bed can improve successful closure of the leak.[62] Prompt identification of a chyle leak in the postoperative setting can help avoid wound complications and anticipate potential metabolic derangements (eg, hyponatremia, hypochloremia, and hypovolemia). Bulb suction (eg, Jackson-Pratt) drains are almost universally placed in the wound bed after extirpative procedures, including neck dissections; sudden appearance of creamy or milky drain output is highly suspicious for a chyle leak. Biochemical confirmation of chyle is made if the drain output tests for a triglyceride level above 100 mg/dL or exceeds the serum triglyceride level.[63] Varying drain output thresholds (500–1000 mL/d) have been reported that are meant to guide clinicians toward nonsurgical management versus intraoperative ligation of the thoracic duct.[64] Given the variability dictating criteria for a high-flow leak, Park and colleagues[61] advocated for nonoperative treatment of chyle leakage for at least 2 days and considering surgical intervention if the drain output had not been reduced by 50% by that time. Conservative treatment of low-flow chyle leaks should include (1) limitations on straining and physical activity to minimize intrathoracic and intraabdominal pressure; (2) medium-chain fatty acid or nonfat diet, with or without concomitant pancreatic lipase inhibitor administration to reduce lipid absorption into the chylous circulation; (3) consideration of pressure dressing or suction drainage, though the clinical benefit of these adjuncts is not definitive; and (4) strong consideration of subcutaneous octreotide, a somatostatin analog, administered (100–200 μg) every 8 hours to 12 hours until resolution of the chyle leak. Octreotide has been a valuable adjunct in the management of chyle, even being sufficient for the treatment of even high-flow leaks after 7 days of administration.[65] Octreotide is proposed to work for chyle leaks by diminishing triglyceride absorption and inhibiting splanchnic circulation and gastrointestinal motility.[66]

Neck hematoma

A recent investigation of major head and neck surgeries revealed that the overall incidence of postoperative neck hematoma was 3.4%, resulting in 540% increased odds of death ($P<.001$) and additional length of stay and excess cost of 5.14 days ($P<.001$) and \$17,887.40 ($P<.001$), respectively.[67] Given the restricted volume of the neck, an expanding, postoperative hematoma can result in acute airway compromise, necessitating prompt evacuation and either surgical or endotracheal airway management. Given the potential rapidity with which compressive hematomas can threaten the patient airway or the vitality of a microvascular free flap, bedside evacuation under local anesthesia sometimes is necessary. Although hematoma formation can complicate any neck procedure, preexisting coagulopathy (hazard ratio 4.15) and free flap reconstruction (hazard ratio 2.28) have been reported as predictors.[67]

SUMMARY

Head and neck surgical patients, at times, can represent a challenging population to manage in the ICU postoperatively. Close interaction between the critical care and surgical teams, awareness of potential surgery specific complications, and utilization of protocol driven care can reduce risk of morbidity significantly in this population and enhance outcomes.

REFERENCES

1. Andel C, Davidow SL, Hollander M, et al. The economics of health care quality and medical errors. J Health Care Finance 2012;39(1):39–50.
2. Agnelli G. Prevention of venous thromboembolism in surgical patients. Circulation 2004;110(24_suppl_1). IV-4–IV-12.
3. Ahmad FI, Clayburgh DR. Venous thromboembolism in head and neck cancer surgery. Cancers Head Neck 2016;1(1). https://doi.org/10.1186/s41199-016-0014-9.
4. Bahl V, Shuman AG, Hu HM, et al. Chemoprophylaxis for venous thromboembolism in otolaryngology. JAMA Otolaryngol Head Neck Surg 2014;140(11):999.
5. Caprini JA. Thrombosis risk assessment as a guide to quality patient care. Dis Mon 2005;51(2–3):70–8.
6. Cramer JD, Shuman AG, Brenner MJ. Antithrombotic therapy for venous thromboembolism and prevention of thrombosis in otolaryngology–head and neck surgery: state of the art review. Otolaryngol Head Neck Surg 2018;158(4):627–36.
7. Bratzler D, Dellinger EP, Olsen K, et al. Clinical practice guidelines for antimicrobial prophylaxis in surgery. Am J Health Syst Pharm 2013;70:195–283.
8. Langerman A, Thisted R, Hohmann S, et al. Antibiotic and duration of perioperative prophylaxis predicts surgical site infection in head and neck surgery. Otolaryngol Head Neck Surg 2016;154(6):1054–63.
9. Vila PM, Zenga J, Jackson RS. Antibiotic prophylaxis in clean-contaminated head and neck surgery: a systematic review and meta-analysis. Otolaryngol Head Neck Surg 2017;157(4):580–8.
10. Yarlagadda BB, Deschler DG, Rich DL, et al. Head and neck free flap surgical site infections in the era of the Surgical Care Improvement Project. Head Neck 2016;38(Suppl 1):E392–8.

11. Pool C, Kass J, Spivack J, et al. Increased surgical site infection rates following clindamycin use in head and neck free tissue transfer. Otolaryngol Head Neck Surg 2016;154(2):272–8.

12. Jethwa AR, Khariwala SS. What is the preferred perioperative antibiotic choice and duration of use following major head and neck surgery? Laryngoscope 2017;127(5):1009–10.

13. Müller-Richter U, Betz C, Hartmann S, et al. Nutrition management for head and neck cancer patients improves clinical outcome and survival. Nutr Res 2017; 48:1–8.

14. Lopez MJ, Robinson P, Madden T, et al. Nutritional support and prognosis in patients with head and neck cancer. J Surg Oncol 1994;55(1):33–6.

15. Peterson GN, Domino KB, Caplan RA, et al. Management of the difficult airway: a closed claims analysis. Anesthesiology 2005;103(1):33–9.

16. Mathew JP, Rosenbaum SH, O'Connor T, et al. Emergency tracheal intubation in the postanesthesia care unit: physician error or patient disease? Anesth Analg 1990;71(6):691–7.

17. Dosemeci L, Yilmaz M, Yegin A, et al. The routine use of pediatric airway exchange catheter after extubation of adult patients who have undergone maxillofacial or major neck surgery: a clinical observational study. Crit Care 2004;8(6): R385–90.

18. Apfelbaum JL, Hagberg CA, Caplan RA, et al. Practice guidelines for management of the difficult airway an updated report by the American Society of Anesthesiologists task force on management of the difficult airway. Anesthesiology 2013; 118(2):251–70.

19. Membership of the Difficult Airway Society Extubation Guidelines Group, Popat M, Mitchell V, Dravid R, et al. Difficult Airway Society guidelines for the management of tracheal extubation: management of tracheal extubation. Anaesthesia 2012;67(3):318–40.

20. Disa JJ, Pusic AL, Hidalgo DH, et al. Simplifying microvascular head and neck reconstruction: a rational approach to donor site selection. Ann Plast Surg 2001;47(4):385–9.

21. Chen K-T, Mardini S, Chuang DC-C, et al. Timing of presentation of the first signs of vascular compromise dictates the salvage outcome of free flap transfers. Plast Reconstr Surg 2007;120(1):187–95.

22. Gao R, Loo S. Review of 100 consecutive microvascular free flaps. N Z Med J 2011;124(1345):49–56.

23. Hyodo I, Nakayama B, Kato H, et al. Analysis of salvage operation in head and neck microsurgical reconstruction. Laryngoscope 2007;117(2):357–60.

24. Pollei TR, Hinni ML, Moore EJ, et al. Analysis of postoperative bleeding and risk factors in transoral surgery of the oropharynx. JAMA Otolaryngol Head Neck Surg 2013;139(11):1212.

25. Kubik M, Mandal R, Albergotti W, et al. Effect of transcervical arterial ligation on the severity of postoperative hemorrhage after transoral robotic surgery. Head Neck 2017;39(8):1510–5.

26. Ramakrishnan VR, Kingdom TT, Nayak JV, et al. Nationwide incidence of major complications in endoscopic sinus surgery. Int Forum Allergy Rhinol 2012; 2(1):34–9.

27. Platt MP, Parnes SM. Management of unexpected cerebrospinal fluid leak during endoscopic sinus surgery. Curr Opin Otolaryngol Head Neck Surg 2009;17(1): 28–32.

28. Ledderose GJ, Stelter K, Betz CS, et al. Cerebrospinal fluid leaks during endoscopic sinus surgery in thirty-two patients. Clin Otolaryngol 2017;42(5):1105–8.
29. Daudia A, Biswas D, Jones NS. Risk of meningitis with cerebrospinal fluid rhinorrhea. Ann Otol Rhinol Laryngol 2007;116(12):902–5.
30. Ahmed OH, Marcus S, Tauber JR, et al. Efficacy of perioperative lumbar drainage following endonasal endoscopic cerebrospinal fluid leak repair: a meta-analysis. Otolaryngol Head Neck Surg 2017;156(1):52–60.
31. Antibiotic prophylaxis for preventing meningitis in patients with basilar skull fractures. Available at: https://reference.medscape.com/medline/abstract/25918919. Accessed March 4, 2019.
32. Ramadan HH, El Solh AA. An update on otolaryngology in critical care. Am J Respir Crit Care Med 2004;169(12):1273–7.
33. Yu M. Tracheostomy patients on the ward: multiple benefits from a multidisciplinary team? Crit Care 2010;14(1):109.
34. Young D, Harrison DA, Cuthbertson BH, et al. Effect of early vs late tracheostomy placement on survival in patients receiving mechanical ventilation: the TracMan randomized trial. JAMA 2013;309(20):2121–9.
35. Plummer AL, Gracey DR. Consensus conference on artificial airways in patients receiving mechanical ventilation. Chest 1989;96(1):178–80.
36. Liu CC, Livingstone D, Dixon E, et al. Early versus late tracheostomy: a systematic review and meta-analysis. Otolaryngol Head Neck Surg 2015;152(2):219–27.
37. Santos PM, Afrassiabi A, Weymuller EA. Risk factors associated with prolonged intubation and laryngeal injury. Otolaryngol Head Neck Surg 1994;111(4):453–9.
38. Colton House J, Noordzij JP, Murgia B, et al. Laryngeal injury from prolonged intubation: a prospective analysis of contributing factors. Laryngoscope 2011;121(3):596–600.
39. Halum SL, Ting JY, Plowman EK, et al. A multi-institutional analysis of tracheotomy complications. Laryngoscope 2012;122(1):38–45.
40. Bogdasarian RS, Olson NR. Posterior glottic laryngeal stenosis. Otolaryngol Head Neck Surg 1980;88(6):765–72.
41. Whited RE. A prospective study of laryngotracheal sequelae in long-term intubation. Laryngoscope 1984;94(3):367–77.
42. Hillel AT, Karatayli-Ozgursoy S, Samad I, et al. Predictors of posterior glottic stenosis: a multi-institutional case-control study. Ann Otol Rhinol Laryngol 2016;125(3):257–63.
43. Manica D, Schweiger C, Maróstica PJC, et al. Association between length of intubation and subglottic stenosis in children: length of intubation and SGS. Laryngoscope 2013;123(4):1049–54.
44. Shah RK, Lander L, Berry JG, et al. Tracheotomy outcomes and complications: a national perspective. Laryngoscope 2012;122(1):25–9.
45. Grant CA, Dempsey G, Harrison J, et al. Tracheo-innominate artery fistula after percutaneous tracheostomy: three case reports and a clinical review. Br J Anaesth 2006;96(1):127–31.
46. Jones JW, Reynolds M, Hewitt RL, et al. Tracheo-innominate artery erosion: successful surgical management of a devastating complication. Ann Surg 1976;184(2):194–204.
47. White AC, Purcell E, Urquhart MB, et al. Accidental decannulation following placement of a tracheostomy tube. Respir Care 2012;57(12):2019–25.
48. Meltzer C, Klau M, Gurushanthaiah D, et al. Surgeon volume in thyroid surgery: surgical efficiency, outcomes, and utilization. Laryngoscope 2016;126(11):2630–9.

49. RULLI F, AMBROGI V, DIONIGI G, et al. Meta-analysis of recurrent laryngeal nerve injury in thyroid surgery with or without intraoperative nerve monitoring. Acta Otorhinolaryngol Ital 2014;34(4):223–9.
50. Bhattacharyya N, Kotz T, Shapiro J. Dysphagia and aspiration with unilateral vocal cord immobility: incidence, characterization, and response to surgical treatment. Ann Otol Rhinol Laryngol 2002;111(8):672–9.
51. Ritter K, Elfenbein D, Schneider D, et al. Hypoparathyroidism after total thyroidectomy: incidence and resolution. J Surg Res 2015;197(2):348–53.
52. Sywak MS, Palazzo FF, Yeh M, et al. Parathyroid hormone assay predicts hypocalcaemia after total thyroidectomy. ANZ J Surg 2007;77(8):667–70.
53. Wang TS, Roman SA, Sosa JA. Postoperative calcium supplementation in patients undergoing thyroidectomy. Curr Opin Oncol 2012;24(1):22–8.
54. Bilezikian JP, Brandi ML, Cusano NE, et al. Management of hypoparathyroidism: present and future. J Clin Endocrinol Metab 2016;101(6):2313–24.
55. Boyce SE, Meyers AD. Oral feeding after total laryngectomy. Head Neck 1989; 11(3):269–73.
56. Macdonald S, Gan J, McKay AJ, et al. Endovascular treatment of acute carotid blow-out syndrome. J Vasc Interv Radiol 2000;11(9):1184–8.
57. Aswani J, Thandar M, Otiti J, et al. Early oral feeding following total laryngectomy. J Laryngol Otol 2009;123(03):333.
58. Guimarães AV, Aires FT, Dedivitis RA, et al. Efficacy of pectoralis major muscle flap for pharyngocutaneous fistula prevention in salvage total laryngectomy: a systematic review. Head Neck 2016;38(Suppl 1):E2317–21.
59. Li RJ, Zhou XC, Fakhry C, et al. Reduction of pharyngocutaneous fistulae in laryngectomy patients by a comprehensive performance improvement intervention. Otolaryngol Head Neck Surg 2015;153(6):927–34.
60. Crumley RL, Smith JD. Postoperative chylous fistula prevention and management. Laryngoscope 1976;86(6):804–13.
61. Park I, Her N, Choe J-H, et al. Management of chyle leakage after thyroidectomy, cervical lymph node dissection, in patients with thyroid cancer. Head Neck 2018; 40(1):7–15.
62. Zeidan S, Delarue A, Rome A, et al. Fibrin glue application in the management of refractory chylous ascites in children. J Pediatr Gastroenterol Nutr 2008;46(4): 478–81.
63. Delaney SW, Shi H, Shokrani A, et al. Management of chyle leak after head and neck surgery: review of current treatment strategies. Int J Otolaryngol 2017. https://doi.org/10.1155/2017/8362874.
64. Schild HH, Strassburg CP, Welz A, et al. Treatment options in patients with chylothorax. Dtsch Arztebl Int 2013;110(48):819–26.
65. Jain A, Singh SN, Singhal P, et al. A prospective study on the role of octreotide in management of chyle fistula neck. Laryngoscope 2015;125(7):1624–7.
66. Swanson MS, Hudson RL, Bhandari N, et al. Use of octreotide for the management of chyle fistula following neck dissection. JAMA Otolaryngol Head Neck Surg 2015;141(8):723–7.
67. Shah-Becker S, Greenleaf EK, Boltz MM, et al. Neck hematoma after major head and neck surgery: risk factors, costs, and resource utilization. Head Neck 2018; 40(6):1219–27.

Anesthesia for Ambulatory and Office-Based Ear, Nose, and Throat Surgery

Leopoldo V. Rodriguez, MD[a,b,c,d],*

KEYWORDS

- Ambulatory • Office-based • Patient selection criteria

KEY POINTS

- *Surgeon-dependent criteria.* Despite equal training and equivalent certification, there are surgeons who are recognized by their peers as being especially capable and whose patients tend to do best.
- *Patient-dependent criteria.* Not all patients in ambulatory surgery are healthy, not all healthy patients are candidates for ambulatory surgery. To decide which patients should have outpatient procedures is easier than to decide which ones should not. I review the most significant medical conditions that can affect decision making.
- *Anesthesia department.* The surgeon must feel comfortable working with the anesthesia team. Good communication and clinical/technical skills based on evidence based medicine improves outcomes.
- *Discharge issues.* Patients who undergo surgery in an Ambulatory Surgery Center (ASC) are required to be discharged in the company of a responsible adult.
- *Pediatric patient selection criteria for outpatient anesthesiology.* Pediatric patient selection criteria for ambulatory surgery can be based on risk factors for unanticipated admission in children after ambulatory surgery.

INTRODUCTION

For the past 2 decades, improvements in surgical techniques, equipment, anesthetic management, and preoperative optimization, have decreased postsurgical complications; this has caused a shift of surgical volume from hospital inpatient settings to ambulatory settings (57% in 1994 to 66% in 2014.).[1,2] At present, 93.4% of procedures involving the ear and 86.9% of procedures involving the nose, mouth, and/or pharynx occur in the outpatient setting.

Disclosure: The authors have nothing to disclose.
[a] Society for Ambulatory Anesthesiology (SAMBA); [b] ASA Committee on Ambulatory Surgical Care; [c] Surgery Center of Aventura, Aventura, FL, USA; [d] Envision Physician Services, 7700 West Sunrise Boulevard, Plantation, FL 33322, USA
* 1199 South Federal Hwy # 392, Boca Raton, FL 33432.
E-mail address: leopoldorodriguez@icloud.com

Otolaryngol Clin N Am 52 (2019) 1157–1167
https://doi.org/10.1016/j.otc.2019.08.012
0030-6665/19/© 2019 Elsevier Inc. All rights reserved.

oto.theclinics.com

PATIENT SELECTION CRITERIA FOR AMBULATORY ANESTHESIOLOGY

Once a decision has been made to operate, the most significant decision is to choose the location where the procedure will be performed. This article aims to help decide if a patient is a candidate for ambulatory or office-based ear, nose, and throat (ENT) procedures.

Procedure-Dependent Criteria

Procedures that may be appropriately performed in an ambulatory surgical center (ASC) or an office-based setting, exclude those that:

- Are expected to need active medical monitoring and overnight inpatient care;
- Generally result in extensive blood loss or involve major blood vessels;
- Are generally emergent or life-threatening in nature;
- Commonly require systemic thrombolytic therapy.[3]

Commonly performed procedures in ambulatory or office-based settings can be classified based on the invasiveness:

Low risk: cerumen removal, flexible laryngoscopy, nasopharyngoscopy, punch biopsy, removal of foreign body, tracheobronchoscopy via tracheostomy.

Low to moderate risk: control of epistaxis, myringotomy with or without tympanostomy tube, nasal polypectomy, sialoendoscopy.

Moderate risk: balloon-assisted sinus dilation, endoscopic nasopharyngeal biopsy; incision and drainage of auricular hematoma, facial or superficial abscess, inferior turbinate reduction.

Moderate to high risk: flexible laryngoscopy with biopsy, injection; functional endoscopic sinus surgery, and cosmetic facial procedures, including blepharoplasty, rhinoplasty, brow lift, and facial resurfacing.

Surgeon-Dependent Criteria

Despite equal training and equivalent certification, there are surgeons who are recognized by their peers as being especially capable and whose patients tend to do best in terms of surgical outcome and lower morbidity and mortality. Birkmeyer and colleagues[4] demonstrated that the surgical skills of a fully trained surgeon have a direct influence on outcomes. Surgeons evaluating videos of other colleagues performing surgery are able to distinguish best to worst surgical ability using a scale of 1 to 5 (ranging from 2.6 to 4.8). The bottom quartile of technical skill was associated with a significantly higher rate of complications (14.5% vs. 5.2%, $P<.001$); higher rates of reoperation (3.4% vs. 1.6%, $P = .01$), readmission within 30 days (6.3% vs. 2.7%, $P<.001$), and return visits to the emergency department (10.2% vs. 3.8%, $P = .004$), when compared with the upper quartile.

Patients treated by high-volume surgeons had lower operative mortality rates for all procedures studied.[5]

Patient-Dependent Criteria

Successful performance of procedures in an ASC and/or office-based setting are highly dependent on proper patient selection. There are many medical conditions that could prevent the patient from having their surgery in an outpatient setting. A key concept is that preoperative testing in low-risk ambulatory surgery has not been demonstrated to affect perioperative care, decrease complications, cancellations, or delays. It is unnecessary to repeat laboratory analysis if there has been no recent change in the patient's condition. Instead, communication with the primary care provider to review the patient's active medical problems, previous medical history, and management are more beneficial than testing.

Patient comorbidities are intrinsic risk factors that can increase the likelihood of perioperative morbidity and mortality; extrinsic factors such as the type of surgery, can also have an impact on patient outcomes. A Canadian study selected from a population of 20,657 patients who underwent ambulatory surgical procedures, and compared patients who required hospital admission to those who did not. After multiple logistic regression analysis to assess factors that were associated with unanticipated admission, the authors found the following risk factors increased the likelihood of unanticipated admission:

- Length of surgery of 1 to 3 hours, but especially over 3 hours
- American Society of Anesthesiologists (ASA) classification III or IV (4-fold increased risk of admission)
- Advanced age, defined as over 80 years (5-fold increased risk of admission)
- Increased body mass index (BMI), defined as over 35 kg/m^2

The ASA classification, advanced age, and increased BMI can be detected in a preoperative evaluation. Several conditions were found to be present in admitted patients but were not direct factors for admission: diabetes, hypertension, ischemic heart disease, psychiatric illness, sleep apnea, and thyroid disease. Procedures lasting longer than 3 hours have been identified in multiple studies as a risk factor for admission.

Factors that were found to have a lower incidence of admission, included: ENT surgery, monitored anesthesia care, and being a current smoker.[6]

AMERICAN SOCIETY OF ANESTHESIOLOGISTS CLASSIFICATION

The ASA has defined a physical status classification to facilitate communication about the health status of a patient, standardize categories for statistical studies, and for uniform interpretation in hospital records; the ASA PS classification it is not an index of operative risk.[7,8]

- ASA PS I: healthy patients, nonsmokers, with minimal alcohol use
- ASA PS II: patients with mild systemic disease. For example, current smokers, social alcohol drinkers, pregnant, obese (BMI = 30 to <40 kg/m^2), well-controlled hypertension, diabetes mellitus, or asthma
- ASA PS III: patients with severe systemic disease. For example, have 1 or more moderate to severe systemic diseases. Poorly controlled diabetes, hypertension, chronic obstructive pulmonary disease, morbid obesity (>40 kg/m^2), active hepatitis, alcohol dependence, implantable pacemaker, moderate reduction of ejection fraction ($\geq$30%), end-stage renal disease (ESRD) undergoing regular dialysis, premature infant postconceptional age $\leq$60 weeks, history of myocardial infarction (MI) ($\geq$3 months), cerebral vascular accident (CVA), transient ischemic attack (TIA), or coronary artery disease (CAD)/stents
- ASA PS IV: patients with severe systemic disease that is a constant threat to life. These include patients who have had a recent (<3 months) history of MI, CVA, TIA, or CAD/stents, ongoing cardiac ischemia or severe valvular dysfunction, severe reduction of ejection fraction (<30%), survival after surgery for those with a left ventricular ejection fraction (LVEF) $\leq$29% is significantly worse than for those with an LVEF >29%), disseminated intravascular coagulation, acute respiratory distress, or ESRD not undergoing regular dialysis
- ASA PS V: patients who are not expected to survive without the operation

- ASA PS VI: patients who have been declared brain dead and whose organs are being harvested

In general, ASA class IV patients should not undergo ambulatory surgery, or ambulatory anesthesia, unless the procedure is superficial and can performed with none or minimal sedation. ASA class III patients should always be evaluated more carefully when considered for ambulatory surgery; this is reaffirmed by a large cohort study at Duke University. Hopkins and colleagues,[9] evaluated over 700,000 elective and emergency procedures performed at over 233 inpatient and outpatient locations within their health care system. Mortality was found to be 0.001% in ASA class I patients; 0.002% in ASA class II patients; 0.035% in ASA class III patients; and 0.319% in ASA class IV patients ($P<.001$).

With regard to office-based settings, patients who are ASA PS I and II are appropriate for office-based surgery. Less-invasive and lower-risk procedures can be performed in ASA class III patients, but the decision to proceed in an outpatient setting should be made jointly by the ENT surgeon and anesthesiologist.

THE AMERICAN COLLEGE OF SURGEONS SURGICAL RISK CALCULATOR

The American College of Surgeons risk calculator provides accurate, validated, patient-specific risk information to guide both surgical decision making and informed consent. The risk calculator uses patient predictors and the planned procedure CPT code to predict the chance that an individual patient will have any 1 of 15 different complication including death within 30 days after surgery. Based on this information, surgeons can determine which patients should undergo more extensive preoperative evaluation.[10] This provides the opportunity to optimize the patient's health status before surgery, which may include blood pressure control, diabetes management, nutritional assessment, frailty assessment, exercise tolerance, smoking cessation, and treatment of hematologic conditions.

FRAILTY

Patients aged 65 years or older, who undergo elective outpatient surgery, should be assessed for frailty. Frailty is a condition or syndrome which results from a multisystem reduction in reserve capacity to the extent that many physiologic systems are close to, or past, the threshold of symptomatic clinical failure. Frailty scores include body shrinkage, weakness, exhaustion, low physical activity, and slowness in the operational definition.[11] As a consequence, the frail patient is at increased risk of disability and death from minor external stresses. Frailty is associated with increased perioperative morbidity in common ambulatory general surgery operations, independent of age, type of anesthesia, and other comorbidities. Surgeons should consider frailty rather than chronologic age when counseling and selecting patients for elective ambulatory surgery.[12] Frailty is a significant risk factor for unplanned admission after elective outpatient surgery (4.9%) versus nonfrail patients (1.9%, $P<.001$). Frail patients are more likely to suffer complications (4.8% vs. 2.6%, $P<.001$). Admission when frailty is present is 2-fold, however, admission when frailty and a complication are present is 48-fold.[13]

Airway Evaluation and Difficult Airway Management

Accurate preoperative prediction of a potential difficult airway or documentation of a previous difficult airway in a surgical setting with experienced providers is a relative contraindication for office-based surgery. During preoperative evaluation there are many criteria that can alert to the difficulty. El-Ganzouri is an airway evaluation scoring system that encompasses several possible factors in airway difficulty (**Table 1**).

A value of 4 or more has a better predictive value for difficult laryngoscopy than a Mallampati classification superior to 2 (level of evidence: 2+).[14]

Six or more points on the El-Ganzouri score (see **Table 1**) should indicate the use of a video laryngoscope or other alternative device.[15]

Table 1
Preoperative prediction of a potential difficult airway scoring system

Feature	0 Points	1 Point (Each)	2 Points (Each)
Body weight (kg)	<90	90–110	>110
Head and neck flexion/extension (°)	>90	80–90	<80
Mouth opening (cm)	>4	<4	
Ability to bite upper lip	Yes	No	
Thyromental distance (cm)	>6.5	6–6.5	<6
Mallampati	I	II	III or IV
History of difficult intubation	None	Questionable	Definite

Adapted from El-Ganzouri et al.[14]

Obesity

The Society for Ambulatory Anesthesia's selection criteria of obese patients undergoing ambulatory surgery[16] indicates that super obese patients (body mass index [BMI] >50 kg/m^2) present increased perioperative complications, significantly increased mortality, and should not undergo ambulatory surgery. Patients with BMI between 40 and 50 kg/m^2 (severe obesity) should be screened for obesity-related comorbidities that could influence the preoperative cardiac risk, such as atherosclerotic cardiovascular disease, heart failure, resistant systemic hypertension, obstructive sleep apnea (OSA), pulmonary hypertension related to sleep apnea and hypoventilation, cardiac arrhythmias (primarily atrial fibrillation), resistant cardiac failure, and deep vein thrombosis; these patients are not candidates for ambulatory surgery.

Physical examination and electrocardiogram may underestimate cardiac dysfunction in obese patients.

Obesity itself along with associated OSA (see below) and hypoventilation, can induce changes in cardiac hemodynamics associated with obesity (including children) may alter left ventricular structure, function, dysrhythmias, and ultimately cause heart failure. After 10 years of severe obesity, the risk of obesity cardiomyopathy increases significantly.[17] Features include diastolic heart failure, and changes in cardiac structure and function that are reversible after substantial weight loss.[18] The American Heart Association (AHA)/American College of Cardiology (ACC) published guidelines for the evaluation of obese patients for noncardiac surgery. There are six known perioperative cardiovascular morbidity risk factors: (1) high-risk surgery; (2) history of coronary heart disease; (3) history of congestive heart failure; (4) history of cerebrovascular disease; (5) preoperative treatment with insulin; and (6) preoperative creatinine levels of greater than 2.0 mg/dL. Obese patients with no risk of coronary heart disease do not require further testing; however, if patients have ≥3 coronary heart disease risk factors or have diagnosed coronary heart disease they may require additional evaluation, medical optimization, or coronary revascularization. In severely obese patients with at least 1 risk factor for CAD or poor exercise tolerance, it is reasonable to obtain a 12-lead electrocardiogram. If it shows right ventricular hypertrophy, one should consider an underling diagnosis of pulmonary hypertension; a left bundle branch block may suggest occult coronary artery disease. If the patient has poor functional capacity and is unable to exercise, a pharmacologic stress test and or imaging technique to assess cardiac function may be indicated depending on the risk of surgery; if the patient has left ventricular systolic dysfunction, the patient may have obesity cardiomyopathy.

Obstructive Sleep Apnea

Patients with OSA are at risk for many complications. Intraoperatively these patients are more likely to have a difficult airway in terms of ventilation (ie, difficult or failed mask ventilation), causing difficulty in maintenance of adequate postoperative oxygen saturation, and are prone to obstruction after extubation, negative pressure pulmonary edema, exacerbation of cardiac conditions, including hypertension, dysrhythmias, myocardial ischemia, infarction, pulmonary hypertension, heart failure, cerebrovascular disorders, prolonged postanesthesia care unit stay, delayed discharge home, unanticipated hospital admission, hypoxic brain injury, and death. The Society for Ambulatory Anesthesiology statement on preoperative selection of adult patients with OSA scheduled for ambulatory surgery divides patients with presumptive or confirmed diagnosis of OSA into 2 groups, those with optimized comorbidities and those with nonoptimized comorbid medical conditions.

Patients with OSA with BMI less than 50 m/kg^2 and optimized comorbid conditions can be considered for ambulatory surgery, as long as the surgeon, patient, and anesthesiologist agree that postoperative pain can be managed predominantly with nonopioid analgesic techniques. Patients with OSA with nonoptimized comorbid medical conditions are not candidates for ambulatory surgery and could benefit from further diagnosis and treatment of comorbidities before surgery.[19] There is insufficient evidence in the current literature to support canceling or delaying surgery for a formal sleep study in patients with suspected OSA; however, preoperative cardiopulmonary optimization should be considered in patients with diagnosed, partially treated/untreated, and suspected OSA where there is indication of an associated significant or uncontrolled systemic disease or additional problems with ventilation or gas exchange, such as hypoventilation syndromes, severe pulmonary hypertension, and resting hypoxemia in the absence of other cardiopulmonary diseases.

PREOPERATIVE CARDIAC EVALUATION

According to the 2014 ACC/AHA Perioperative Clinical Practice Guideline, ENT procedures without planned flap or neck dissection are associated with minimal physiologic effects, and thus are considered low-risk surgery. What really matters for elective outpatient surgery are good functional capacity and that patients are medically optimized from the cardiopulmonary point of view. For example, a patient with hypertension and blood pressure of 140/90 mm Hg may be considered optimized by the primary care physician; however, this may not be an optimal blood pressure for sinus surgery because of the risk of intraoperative and postoperative bleeding. It is important to know that intraoperative decrease in blood pressure in either systolic or mean arterial blood pressure, have been identified as a risk factor for complications, such as acute kidney injury, cardiac injury, postoperative neurologic dysfunction, and death; thus, intraoperative hemodynamics should aim to maintain the blood pressure within ±10% of the baseline blood pressure; and to keep intraoperative mean arterial pressure (MAP) greater than 65 mm Hg (increased mortality when mean arterial pressure is <55%.)[20] Holding angiotensin-converting enzyme inhibitors and angiotensin II receptor blockers on the day of surgery reduces intraoperative hypotension and the risk of death, myocardial injury after noncardiac surgery, or stroke by about 20%, and over 500,000 patients per year would avoid death or stroke within 30 days of their operation.[21]

In 2011, the Heart Rhythm Society and other societies published the guidelines for management of cardiac implantable electronic devices, also known as pacemakers and defibrillators. Patients with cardiac implantable electronic devices are classified as ASA PS III, and can undergo ambulatory surgery. The Heart Rhythm Society guidelines publish a process to be followed to manage patients in any setting. In brief, when a procedure can be performed without electromagnetic interference, one should only check the battery life and proper device function within the previous month. If electromagnetic interference is to be used, and if the procedure is within 15 cm or 6 inches of the device, then additional precautions should be taken, including application of a magnet to prevent the artifact being interpreted as a tachydysrhythmia or device inhibition; the cardiologist can also suggest to change the program to asynchronous mode or eliminate physiologic programming. It is recommended that the facility and anesthesiologist be advised of the device, good communication with the patient's cardiologist prevents unnecessary cancellations. The Heart Rhythm Society included a list of reasons for the device to be checked before discharge.[22]

Dual Antiplatelet Therapy

In 2016, the AHA/ACC published an update for the use of dual antiplatelet therapy (DAPT)[23] after cardiac stenting or coronary artery bypass graft. Patients who suffered an acute coronary syndrome with ST-segment elevation myocardial infarction, and who underwent coronary artery bypass graft or percutaneous coronary intervention with a drug-eluting stent should remain on DAPT for 12 months. Patients who did not have an acute coronary syndrome but instead were diagnosed with coronary artery disease and an elective coronary artery bypass graft or percutaneous coronary intervention with drug-eluting stents should remain for 6 months on DAPT. For newer-generation drug-eluting stents (fourth generation), the temporary scaffold that safeguards vessel patency, which disappears, is presently the ideal solution for treating CAD. These fourth-generation stents allow the vessel to potentially restore its vascular function (vessel vasomotion), adaptive shear stress, late luminal enlargement, and remodeling.

- Patients who receive a bare metal stent should continue DAPT for at least 1 month.
- Patients with cardiac stents should remain on aspirin 81 mg/day for life unless contraindicated and need to remain on aspirin during the perioperative period for all ENT surgeries.

Because mortality remains higher if DAPT treatment is continued for less than 6 months, it is our recommendation that those procedures should be performed in a center capable of performing a cardiac catheterization, because acute in-stent thrombosis has a very high mortality rate.
The risk of significant bleeding when continuing DAPT is higher than 6.7%.

DIABETES

In 2019, the American Diabetes Association recommends to check hemoglobin A_{1C} within the 30 days before surgery, with a target hemoglobin A_{1C} of less than 8.5% in most nonpregnant patients with diabetes. However, there is no specific value at which a case should be canceled. A patient's clinical and physiologic status can be evaluated the day of surgery and the decision to proceed or not should be made by the ENT surgeon and the anesthesiologist. In the perioperative setting, pharmacologic therapy can be initiated for hyperglycemia consistently more than 140 mg/dL. Insulin therapy should be initiated for persistent hyperglycemia more than 180 mg/d. Target blood glucose is between 140 and 180 mg/dL to prevent episodes of hypoglycemia.[24]

The Society for Ambulatory Anesthesiology consensus statement for the management of diabetic patients undergoing elective ambulatory surgery gives specific recommendations for the preoperative dosage of medications to manage diabetes.[25–27]

Other hematologic conditions should be discussed with the patient, hematologist, anesthesiologist, and facility staff to plan a safe perioperative period for the patient. There may be medication or biological factors that are not available at an ASC and thus may require the procedure to be performed at a hospital.

Stroke and Transient Ischemic Attacks

Jorgensen and colleagues[28] recommend delaying elective surgical procedures for 9 months after an ischemic stroke to prevent major adverse cardiovascular events, mortality, and a repeat stroke. Amarenco and colleagues[29] followed 4583 patients after a TIA diagnosed by a neurologist and found that, at 1 year, 25 died from cardiovascular causes, 210 suffered nonfatal stroke, and 39 a nonfatal acute coronary syndrome. After analyzing the data, based on $ABCD^2$ score, those patients with a score of 0 to 3 had increased risk until approximately 3 months post-TIA; those with a score of 4 to 5 had increased risk until 6 to 9 months post-TIA; and those with a score of 6 to 7 maintained a high risk of recurrent stroke for over 9 months.

Facility-Dependent Criteria

There is considerable evidence that patients being treated or undergoing procedures have lower mortality rates and better outcomes if care is provided in facilities with a high caseload of patients with the same condition when compared with institutions with a lower case load.[5] When considering a facility, the surgeon must consider the ability of the staff, surgical equipment instrument availability, the quality of the postanesthesia care unit, and the availability of emergency equipment.

Discharge Issues

Patients who undergo surgery in an ASC are required to be discharged in the company of a responsible adult. We recommend that patients who receive medications that alter their mental status or have a procedure that limit the patient's ability to take care of themselves remain with an adult caretaker. The risk of falls and postoperative confusion caused by medications must be considered.

Patient Selection Criteria for Office-Based Anesthesiology

Patient exclusion criteria for office-based surgery include: ASA PS class 3 or 4 patients with history of substance abuse, poorly controlled medical comorbidities, seizure disorder, morbid obesity, OSA, extremes of life (in Florida 13 years or older), no responsible adult escort. The ASA recommends that patients who are American

Society for Anesthesiologists Physical Status I and II are suitable candidates for office-based Anesthesiology. Patients who are American Society for Anesthesiologists Physical Status III should have a consultation with the anesthesiologist before the day of the procedure to decide if they are a candidate for office-based surgery.

PEDIATRIC PATIENT SELECTION CRITERIA FOR OUTPATIENT ANESTHESIOLOGY
Children Are Not Small Adults

Pediatric patient selection criteria for ambulatory surgery can be based on risk factors for unanticipated admission of children after ambulatory surgery. These include anesthesia-related events, age less than 2 years, ASA PS III; duration of surgery more than 1 h, surgical procedure after 3 PM, orthopedic, dental, and ENT surgery, intraoperative-events, and OSA were statistically significant factors predictive of unanticipated admission.[30]

Nationwide Children's Hospital pediatric adenotonsillectomy guidelines help decide which patients should undergo surgery in an ASC versus a hospital setting. Patients who should be operated in a hospital include those for a tonsillectomy at an age less than 3 years, or age less than 2 years for adenoidectomy, craniofacial disorders, and comorbid conditions such as hypotonia, cystic fibrosis, heart disease, hematologic disorders, diabetes mellitus, or uncontrolled asthma. Pediatric patients with confirmed OSA by polysomnography should be treated as inpatients if their apnea hypopnea index is greater than 10 episodes per hour, their end tidal CO_2 is greater than 50 mm Hg, and they have an oxygen nadir of less than 80%.[31]

SUMMARY: PRIMUM NON NOCERE

A good physician treats the disease; a great physician treats the patient who has the disease
> *—Moses Maimonides (Rambam) in his Treatise on Asthma*

As anesthesiology has evolved with newer shorter-acting medications with less side effects, and surgical equipment and techniques have improved, we must take a holistic approach, and carefully select which surgeons, procedures, anesthesiologists, allied health providers, facilities, and patients should be involved in ambulatory and office-based surgery.

As described, selection criteria for each of the above key points has a better and direct correlation with patient outcomes and quality of care.

REFERENCES

1. American Hospital Association. Utilization and Volume. Trends Affecting Hospitals and Health Systems. Updated for 2016; chapter 3. Available at: https://www.aha.org/system/files/research/reports/tw/chartbook/2016/chapter3.pdf Accessed September 12, 2019.
2. Steiner CA (Institute for Health Research, Kaiser Permanente), Karaca Z (AHRQ), Moore BJ (IBM Watson Health), Imshaug MC (IBM Watson Health), Pickens G (IBM Watson Health). Surgeries in hospital-based ambulatory surgery and hospital inpatient settings, 2014. HCUP statistical brief #223. Rockville (MD): Agency for Healthcare Research and Quality; 2017. Available at: www.hcup-us.ahrq.gov/reports/statbriefs/sb223-Ambulatory-Inpatient-Surgeries-2014.pdf. Accessed September 12, 2019.

3. American Academy of Otolaryngology—Head and Neck Surgery. Position statement: Ambulatory procedures. Available at: http://www.entnet.org/content/ambulatory-procedures. Accessed September 12, 2019.

4. Birkmeyer JD, Finks JF, O'Reilly A, et al. Surgical skill and complication rates after bariatric surgery. N Engl J Med 2013;369:1434–42.

5. Birkmeyer JD, Siewers AE, Finlayson EV, et al. Hospital volume and surgical mortality in the United States. N Engl J Med 2002;346:1128–37.

6. Whippey A, Kostandoff G, Paul J, et al. Predictors of unanticipated admission following ambulatory surgery: a retrospective case-control study. Can J Anaesth 2013;60:675–83.

7. ASA Physical Status Classification System. Developed by ASA House of Delegates/Executive Committee. Last amended: October 15, 2014 (original approval: October 15, 2014). Available at: https://www.asahq.org/standards-and-guidelines/asa-physical-status-classification-system. Accessed September 12, 2019.

8. Owens W, Felts J, Spitznagel E. ASA physical status classifications: a study of consistency of ratings. Anesthesiology 1978;49:239–43.

9. Hopkins T, Raghunathan K, Barbeito A, et al. Associations between ASA Physical Status and postoperative mortality at 48 h: a contemporary dataset analysis compared to a historical cohort. Perioper Med (Lond) 2016;5:29.

10. Available at: www.riskcalculator.facs.org/. Accessed September 12, 2019.

11. Makary M, Segev DL, Pronovost PJ, et al. Frailty as a predictor of surgical outcomes in older patients. J Am Coll Surg 2010;210:901–8.

12. Seib CD, Rochefort H, Chomsky-Higgins K, et al. Association of patient frailty with increased morbidity after common ambulatory general surgery operations. JAMA Surg 2018;153(2):160–8.

13. Stern J, Blum K, Trickey A, et al. Interaction of frailty and postoperative complications on unplanned readmission after elective outpatient surgery. J Am Coll Surg 2018;227(4, Suppl 2):25.

14. El-Ganzouri AR, McCarthy RJ, Tuman KJ, et al. Preoperative airway assessment: predictive value of a multivariate risk index. Anesth Analg 1996;82:1197–204.

15. Cortellazzi P, Minati L, Falcone C, et al. Predictive value of the El-Ganzouri multivariate risk index for difficult tracheal intubation: a comparison of Glidescope videolaryngoscopy and conventional Macintosh laryngoscopy. Br J Anaesth 2007;99(6):906–11.

16. Joshi G, Ahmad S, Riad W, et al. Society for Ambulatory Anesthesiology, selection of obese patients undergoing ambulatory surgery: a systematic review of the literature. Anesth Analg 2013;117:1082–91.

17. Poirier P, Alpert MA, Fleisher LA, et al. Cardiovascular evaluation and management of severely obese patients undergoing surgery: a science advisory from the American Heart Association. Circulation 2009;120:86–95.

18. Timoh T, Bloom ME, Siegel R, et al. A perspective on obesity cardiomyopathy. Obes Res Clin Pract 2012;6(3):e181–8.

19. Joshi G, Ankichetty S, Gan TJ, et al. Society for Ambulatory Anesthesia consensus statement on preoperative selection of adult patients with obstructive sleep apnea scheduled for ambulatory surgery. Anesth Analg 2012;115:1060–8.

20. Walsh M, Devereaux P, Garg A, et al. Relationship between intraoperative mean arterial pressure and clinical outcomes after noncardiac surgery: toward an empirical definition of hypotension. Anesthesiology 2013;119:507–13.

21. Roshaov P, Rochwerg B, Patel A, et al. Withholding versus continuing angiotensin-converting enzyme inhibitors or angiotensin II receptor blockers

before noncardiac surgery: an analysis of the vascular events in noncardiac surgery patients cohort evaluation prospective cohort. Anesthesiology 2017;126: 16–27.

22. Crossley GH, Poole JE, Rozner MA, et al. The Heart Rhythm Society (HRS)/American Society of Anesthesiologists (ASA) Expert Consensus Statement on the perioperative management of patients with implantable defibrillators, pacemakers and arrhythmia monitors: facilities and patient management: executive summary this document was developed as a joint project with the American Society of Anesthesiologists (ASA), and in collaboration with the American Heart Association (AHA), and the Society of Thoracic Surgeons (STS). Heart Rhythm 2011;8(7): E1–18.

23. Levine GN, Bates ER, Bittl JA, et al. 2016 ACC/AHA guideline focused update on duration of dual antiplatelet therapy in patients with coronary artery disease. A report of the American College of Cardiology/American Heart Association Task Force on clinical practice guidelines focused update on duration of dual antiplatelet therapy. Circulation 2016;133:e123–55.

24. American Diabetes Association. 15. Diabetes care in the hospital: standards of medical care in diabetes 2019. Diabetes Care 2019;42(Suppl. 1):S173–81.

25. Joshi G, Chung F, Vann M, et al. Society for ambulatory anesthesia consensus statement on perioperative blood glucose management in diabetic patients undergoing ambulatory surgery. Anesth Analg 2010;111:1378–87.

26. Society of Ambulatory Anesthesia (SAMBA). Consensus Statement on Perioperative Blood Glucose Management in Diabetic Patients Undergoing Ambulatory Surgery. Anesth Analg 2010;111(6):1378–87.

27. Korpman T. Review of the consensus statement and additional commentary California Society of Anesthesiologists. Available at: http://www.csahq.org/docs/default-source/news-and-events-docs/csa-bulletin-docs/fall-2010/v59_4_samba_consensus.pdf?sfvrsn=a4f0c646_2. Accessed September 12, 2019.

28. Jorgensen ME, Torp-Pedersen C, Gislason GH, et al. Time elapsed after ischemic stroke and risk of adverse cardiovascular events and mortality following elective noncardiac surgery. JAMA 2014;312(3):269–77.

29. Amarenco P, Lavallée PC, Labreuche J, et al. One-year risk of stroke after transient ischemic attack or minor stroke. N Engl J Med 2016;374:1533–42.

30. Whippey A, Kostandoff G, Ma HK, et al. Predictors of unanticipated admission following ambulatory surgery in the pediatric population: a retrospective case-control study. Paediatr Anaesth 2016;(26):831–7.

31. Raman VT, Jatana KR, Elmaraghy CA, et al. Guidelines to decrease unanticipated hospital admission following adenotonsillectomy in the pediatric population. Int J Pediatr Otorhinolaryngol 2014;78(1):19–22.

Printed and bound by CPI Group (UK) Ltd, Croydon, CR0 4YY

08/05/2025

01864746-0008